Ambivalence in Psychotherapy

Ambivalence in Psychotherapy

FACILITATING READINESS TO CHANGE

David E. Engle
Hal Arkowitz

The Guilford Press
New York   London

© 2006 The Guilford Press
A Division of Guilford Publications, Inc.
72 Spring Street, New York, NY 10012
www.guilford.com

Printed in the United States of America

This book is printed on acid-free paper.

Last digit is print number: 9   8   7   6   5   4   3   2   1

Library of Congress Cataloging-in-Publication Data is available from
the Publisher.

ISBN 1-59385-255-X

*To my wife, Jeanne, and to the members
of the Columbia, Missouri, gestalt training group*
—DEE

*To my children, Laura, Jenny, and Alex,
and my grandchildren, Mackenzie and Sarah*
—HA

About the Authors

David E. Engle, PhD, is a therapist in private practice in Tucson, Arizona, and has been an instructor in gestalt and experiential psychotherapy for many years. Interested in both research and clinical practice, he has published numerous articles and is a coauthor of *Focused Expressive Psychotherapy.* Dr. Engle has been a summer faculty member at the University of Arizona's Division of Education and Professional Studies, and served for 5 years as Projects Coordinator for the Arizona Psychotherapy Project, University of Arizona College of Medicine, Tucson.

Hal Arkowitz, PhD, is Associate Professor of Psychology at the University of Arizona, Tucson, and has researched and published actively in the areas of anxiety, depression, and psychotherapy. He also maintains a clinical practice. Dr. Arkowitz was Editor of the *Journal of Psychotherapy Integration* for 10 years and has coedited two books: *Comprehensive Handbook of Cognitive Therapy* and *Psychoanalytic and Behavior Therapy: Toward an Integration.*

Preface

Ambivalence is a basic human experience. Our wishes and desires lead us to approach our goals, while our fears and concerns lead us to avoid them. The net result is a vacillation that often paralyzes us and prevents us from making changes that would improve our lives.

Surprisingly, ambivalence has received relatively little attention in research and clinical work. We believe that ambivalence is an extremely valuable construct for clinical psychology that can help us understand why people change and why they don't. Furthermore, we believe that working with people to help them resolve ambivalence can significantly facilitate positive change. Once ambivalence is resolved, the work of change proceeds more easily. For these reasons, we decided to write a book on understanding and working with ambivalence to facilitate change.

While the construct of ambivalence has been relatively neglected, other constructs such as resistance and noncompliance have been much more visible in the literature. However, instead of trying to address why people "resist" change, we have posed the issue more broadly with the question "Why don't people change?" This question doesn't carry the pejorative or theoretical baggage associated with the terms "resistance" or "noncompliance," and allowed us to search widely for answers. One major conclusion that we arrived at was that many of the phenomena that are referred to as "resistance" can be better understood as ambivalence. As a result, we have tried to inform readers about the nature of resistance by recasting it as ambivalence.

Resistance and change aren't just flip sides of the same coin. *Resistance* is an active and conflictual process that most often involves the desire for change as well as impediments to change. We believe that understanding and working with client ambivalence can be a crucial aspect of helping people change.

In the tradition of psychotherapy integration, we have looked for common ground among the different theories that attempt to understand and work with ambivalence and resistance, as well as these theories' unique contributions. It may be that each of the theories sees one part of the elephant, but the whole elephant still eludes us. Our approach to resistance is an attempt to see the whole elephant, but we sincerely hope that it won't be referred to as the "whole-elephant approach." We prefer to call it an "integrative approach," and we hope that clinicians and researchers alike will find this book helpful.

Acknowledgments

We are eager to acknowledge a number of people who have greatly influenced our understanding of psychotherapy and change. Their wisdom is reflected in the pages of this book.

Leslie Greenberg's work has been a major influence on our thinking and on this book. He has creatively combined the accepting style of the client-centered therapy of Carl Rogers with experientially oriented gestalt therapy. He has also helped move the field of psychotherapy research toward a deeper understanding of in-session therapy processes. He and his colleagues have provided a much-needed research base for experiential psychotherapy. We read his work on internal conflicts and two-chair work with particular interest. It was enormously helpful in understanding resistance as an internal conflict and inspired us to use the two-chair method as one of our main strategies for working with resistance.

I (DEE) am also indebted to Marjorie Holiman, a talented colleague with whom I have had the privilege of working for more than 20 years. Our collaboration has helped me learn how to understand the subtleties of experiential psychotherapy and how to effectively teach others to be skilled experiential practitioners. Marjorie has an uncanny knack for tweaking our teaching methods to meet the needs of each training group and each individual in those groups.

I (HA) would like to express my deep appreciation to Paul Wachtel and Marvin Goldfried for the inspiration and intellectual mentorship they have provided me through their thinking and their work in psychotherapy integration. Their willingness to think beyond the schools of therapy in which they were trained to see what can be learned from other ways of thinking has been a model of intellectual openness for me. It has led me to think integratively about people and change. That thinking is at the heart of this book, and their influence can be seen throughout it.

Another very important influence on my (HA) thinking and on this book has been the work of William R. Miller. Bill has been my student, my friend, and my teacher. His creative work on motivational interviewing, in collaboration with Stephen Rollnick, has been a profound influence on my thinking and on the ideas developed in this book. In addition to being a stellar researcher, Bill is also one of the most deeply respectful and caring people I've ever met. His understanding of people and change, and his compassion, are reflected in the motivational interviewing approach, which I believe has a great deal to offer to helping people change.

Finally, Jim Nageotte, Senior Editor at The Guilford Press, has shepherded this book to its current state. Our first draft had a much narrower focus. Jim wisely encouraged us to "think bigger" and broaden the scope of the book. His input has been creative, and has always been given in a gentle and encouraging manner. We're deeply indebted to him for his contribution to this book.

Contents

Ambivalence in Psychotherapy

CHAPTER 1

An Overview of Resistance and Ambivalence

Resistance to change is a central concept in the field of psychotherapy. Each therapy approach has a somewhat different view of what constitutes resistance, how to best conceptualize it, and how to work with it. As a result of this fragmentation, we are left with a situation in which resistance is one of the most important yet least understood constructs in psychotherapy and change.

Practitioners can turn to a few sources of clinical wisdom to guide them (e.g., Anderson & Stewart, 1983; Ellis, 2002; Leahy, 2001; Strean, 1990). However, most books on the topic are based on clinical observations and are usually closely tied to a specific theory of therapy. There is neither a body of research nor an integrative theory that can guide the work of psychotherapists, regardless of their theoretical preferences.

Resistance is also a major problem in health psychology and behavioral medicine, where it is usually referred to as "noncompliance" or "nonadherence." When one examines theories of noncompliance, one finds some overlap with theories of resistance in psychotherapy. However, there are also considerable differences and work from the areas of health and behavioral medicine rarely informs thinking about resistance in psychotherapy and vice versa. Those who write about resistance to self-directed changes refer to failures in self-control or self-regulation. Fragmentation both within and across these different areas is the rule rather than the exception, with theories and findings from one area rarely informing those of the others. An integrative framework that draws from different viewpoints within and across these fields may advance the field. One purpose of this book is to present such a framework.

We believe that it is more useful to ask the question "Why don't people change?" than to ask "What causes resistance?" The word *resistance* is so laden with different meanings that it is impossible to answer the question without specifying a theoretical context. By contrast, asking "Why don't people change?" allows us to search more broadly among different theories for integrative answers.

So, why don't people change? Prochaska and Prochaska (1999) have suggested that in some instances they simply don't want to change. While determining volition is often a tricky issue (e.g., are they failing to change because they don't want to, or are they saying they don't want to because they haven't been able to?), it is often the case that some people just do not have an intrinsic desire to change, even though others may desire them to change.

Prochaska and Prochaska (1999) further suggest that in many cases people don't change because they just don't know how to change. People may be unaware of effective change strategies (e.g., exposure therapies for anxiety disorders) and may turn instead to ineffective or untested strategies, such as those advertised in the media (e.g., stop smoking and weight reduction programs), expecting success but finding failure. Some medical and mental health professionals may not keep up with the literature in their fields and may be unaware of recently developed effective treatments. In these instances, the best way to facilitate change is to direct the person toward more effective change methods when they are available.

To these two, we add a third reason for people not changing: ambivalence. In many cases, people both want to change and have reservations about changing. In ambivalence, movement toward change is accompanied or followed by movement away from change and toward the status quo. Whether or not change occurs, the degree of change, and how well the change is maintained depends on the balance of the pros and cons of change. *Our main focus in this book is on those instances of resistance that involve ambivalence.*

DEFINITIONS

We use the term "resistance" to refer to behaviors that interfere with making progress toward desired changes. Resistance may occur in the context of the therapeutic relationship, in the relationship with other health-care providers, or to self-directed efforts to change. We define *resistant ambivalence* as a subset of resistance in which there are movements toward change as well as movements away from change. Since most of the literature doesn't distinguish between resistance and ambivalence, we will refer primarily to resistance in this chapter and the next which reviews relevant research and theory. Then, in Chapter 3 and the rest of the book, we will refer to "resistant ambivalence."

MANIFESTATIONS OF RESISTANCE AND AMBIVALENCE

Ambivalence may be about change itself or about the methods to achieve change. A person might realize that a change will lead to less distress and to a better quality of life, but he or she may also believe that change will be accompanied by higher expectations from him- or herself and from others. For example, a client with agoraphobia may be aware that overcoming the problem will lead to greater comfort and personal freedom, but at the same time he or she may fear giving up his or her dependency on significant others.

There may also be ambivalence concerning the methods to achieve change. For example, the same person with agoraphobia may also be ambivalent about exposure therapy. On the one hand, he or she may believe it is the most potentially helpful therapy but, on the other, may not wish to experience the discomfort that is inherent in such treatment: having to approach rather than avoid situations that cause anxiety.

Ambivalence represents an approach–avoidance conflict (Dollard & Miller, 1950) in which change or the methods used to achieve it evoke both approach and avoidance tendencies. More specifically, we suggest that ambivalence involves the following elements:

1. Belief that the change will overall improve the quality of one's life.
2. Belief that one knows what needs to be done in order to accomplish the change.
3. Behaviors indicative of one's movement toward change. These may consist of statements about the desire to change and overt efforts to accomplish the change.
4. Behaviors indicative of one's movement away from change. These may include statements negating or qualifying the desire

to change (e.g., "It's not worth the effort to make the change"; "Yes, I want to change, but . . . "), little effort directed toward change, or engagement in behaviors that interfere with achieving the change.

5. Negative emotional reactions to not changing.

Ambivalence is common when a person is trying to eliminate addictive behaviors (e.g., use of alcohol, drugs, or cigarettes). While people may say that they want to change and try to decrease or to eliminate their addictive behaviors, they often oscillate between change and no change. Many "fall off the wagon" and climb back on again numerous times before they achieve success. Mahoney (1991) has suggested that personal change occurs in an oscillating manner rather than in a smooth progression. These oscillations usually indicate ambivalence. Therapists from all orientations are aware that change is often erratic and marked by progressions and regressions. This is the case whether the change involves specific behaviors, cognitions, views of oneself, or greater awareness or understanding of oneself. To the extent that we can identify this ambivalence and help people resolve it, we will be able to improve the effectiveness of our therapies.

Resistance and ambivalence are significant phenomena in all areas of our lives. In the remainder of this chapter, we focus on the behaviors that define it and how it occurs in the areas of psychotherapy, health care, and self-directed change.

RESISTANCE AND AMBIVALENCE IN PSYCHOTHERAPY

Therapists of every orientation have encountered people who seek out their help; spend time, spend money, and exert effort to receive that help; and yet often act in ways that seem to sabotage the help that they are seeking. They may behave uncooperatively and even antagonistically toward the therapist, they may frequently cancel or come late for sessions, or they may terminate therapy prematurely. All these actions may be due to ambivalent feelings about change, the therapist, the therapy, or poor rapport between the client and the therapist.

We infer resistant ambivalence when clients continue in therapy while not cooperating with the therapist to achieve their goals. For example, Orlinsky, Grawe, and Parks (1994) reviewed a large number of studies of different types of therapy and found strong negative correlations between measures of defensiveness and lack of cooperation, on the one hand, and poor therapy outcomes, on the other. In cognitive and cognitive-behavioral therapy, between-session assignments and experiments are important aspects of treatment. Numerous studies have demonstrated that client noncompliance is associated with poor therapy outcome, In their meta-analysis of 27 studies, Kazantzis, Deane, and Ronan (2000) found that homework compliance was a significant predictor of therapy outcome. Behavioral therapists have commented on the widespread noncompliance they often see in their work that limits the actual effectiveness of these techniques. For example, Marks (1992) commented that while behavioral therapy has a high success rate for those who complete it, approximately 25% of his clients who are suitable for behavioral therapy either refuse to start treatment or start it and drop out prematurely before they've had a chance to try it properly.

Not only are rates of noncompliance high, but reports of compliance may often be inflated. For example, Taylor, Agras, Schneider, and Allen (1983) trained hypertensive clients in relaxation and gave them a relaxation tape and a tape player to use for practice at home. While 80% of the clients reported that they had practiced as often as instructed, a device hidden in the tape recorder revealed that only 40% had actually done so.

When people seek therapy and then terminate prematurely, we can also infer that resistant ambivalence is involved. Phillips (1985) reported that 70% of clients who seek psychotherapy in an outpatient clinic setting drop out of therapy by the third session. Many of these people are probably ambivalent about treatment. In controlled outcome research where clients are monitored more closely, dropout rates are still substantial. For example, Westen and Morrison (2001) reviewed 34 therapy outcome studies on depression, panic disorder, and generalized anxiety disorder and found that dropout rates were 26%, 14%, and 16%, respectively.

BEHAVIORS ASSOCIATED WITH RESISTANCE AND AMBIVALENCE IN PSYCHOTHERAPY

Cavender and Arkowitz (1999) developed a verbal coding system for resistance that can be applied to different therapeutic orientations. Their categories are presented in Table 1.1.

TABLE 1.1. Verbal Indicators of Resistance to Change

Ambivalence

Statements that suggest that the client is pulled in two rather different directions on a particular issue. The classic "yes, but . . . " is an example of this.

Avoidance

Own agenda or sidetrack: These are statements that are not in response to the therapist's questions or interventions, but take off on a different track without any acknowledgment of that fact.

Refusal: Statements in which the client directly refuses an invitation or suggestion or interpretation on the part of the therapist. (Note that such refusal may be quite adaptive and not resistant if the therapist's intervention was a poor one).

Defensiveness: Statements that reflect reluctance to consider therapist comments or questions that are of potential value to the client. These are often accompanied by other statements reflecting disagreement with the therapist's comments.

Helplessness

Inability due to helplessness or hopelessness: Statements that reflect the client's perceived inability ("I can't") to respond to the therapist's intervention (examine a feeling, deal with an issue, try something between sessions, etc.) due to a sense of perceived helplessness or hopelessness.

Note. From Cavender and Arkowitz (1999). Reprinted by permission of the authors.

The reader might react to some of the items by thinking "That's not resistance." We believe that such a reaction is due to the fact that judgments as to what constitutes resistance are relative both to the context in which the behavior occurs and the theoretical orientation from which it is viewed.

The questions of what constitutes resistance and how to conceptualize it become more complicated when we answer those questions from different theoretical perspectives. Because of their very natures, some client behaviors indicative of resistance are more likely to occur in some types of therapy than in others. For example, refusal to follow through with homework assignments would likely be seen often in cognitive-behavioral therapy in which homework assignments are a frequent component, but would rarely be seen in psychodynamic therapy in which such assignments are seldom used. Misinterpretations of the therapist's remarks are more likely to occur in psychodynamic approaches in which the therapist's interpretive comments are central, but perhaps less likely to occur in cognitive-behavioral therapy in which the therapist primarily uses questions rather than interpretations. A major goal of this book is to provide an integrative framework that can subsume resistance from different psychotherapies.

RESISTANCE AND AMBIVALENCE IN MEDICINE AND HEALTH CARE

Physicians and other health care providers are familiar with the phenomenon of people suffering from serious illnesses who come to them for help yet don't sufficiently follow through on the help that they offer. Studies have found that between 50 and 65% of patients do not adhere appropriately to their medication regimen (e.g., Haynes, Taylor, & Sackett, 1979; Schaub, Steiner, & Vetter, 1993). Schlenk, Dunbar-Jacob, and Engberg (2004) report that half of gerontological patients do not comply with medical regimens and that 10% of hospital admissions are the result of medication nonadherence. Van Eijken, Tsang, Wensing, de Smet, and Grol (2003) looked at compliance in people over 60 and found that noncompliance varies from 29 to 59%. Compliance with long-term treatment for asymptomatic conditions such as hypertension is approximately 50% (Loghman-Adham, 2003). Sackett (1976) estimated that between 20 and 50% of physician appointments are missed. Poor compliance is found even when the cost of the program is relatively low and side effects are relatively minimal (cf. Meichenbaum & Turk, 1987; Vincent, 1971). Noncompliance with physicians' recommendations to exercise, lose weight, and stop smoking (Brownell, Marlatt, Lichtenstein, & Wilson, 1986) is particularly high.

   Adherence to medical regimens varies depending on the form of treatment. The highest rates of adherence occur for treatments involving direct medications (e.g., injections or chemotherapy), high levels of supervision or monitoring, and acute onset. The lowest rates of adherence seem to occur for chronic disorders where no immediate risk or discomfort is experienced, when lifestyle changes are required, and when prevention rather than symptom reduction is the desired outcome (Meichenbaum & Turk, 1987).

We should note that while many instances of noncompliance reflect resistant ambivalence, many others do not. For example, a patient who cannot afford the prescribed recommendation will be noncompliant, but not necessarily ambivalent about taking the medication. Many cases of noncompliance in health care are the result of impaired ability that may be due to lack of financial resources, neurological or cognitive deficits that interfere with proper adherence, and even anxiety and depression (see DiMatteo, Lepper, & Croghan, 2000). In addition, studies confirm that poor communication between the health care worker and the patient account for a great deal of noncompliance (DiMatteo, 1993; DiMatteo, Reiter, & Gambone, 1994).

In many areas of medicine, the problem is not the lack of effective treatments, but how to help people carry out existing treatments. If we can help patients resolve their ambivalence and increase their compliance, the effectiveness of treatments in many areas would almost double. While the search for new treatments is important, there is still a great deal of unused potential in existing treatments if we can solve the problem of noncompliance or nonadherence with medical programs. There is no question that the effectiveness of many areas of medicine (e.g., treatment of diabetes and hypertension) would be dramatically increased if patients with those illnesses carried out the treatments diligently.

A particularly dramatic example of noncompliance can be found in a study by Vincent (1971) who interviewed glaucoma patients who were coming for treatment to a community medical clinic. Glaucoma is a progressive disease that if untreated leads to blindness. Effective treatment is readily available in the form of eyedrops, which can prevent the further progress of the disease. The drops need to be administered two to three times a day, and their only side effect is a few minutes of mildly unpleasant burning sensations in the eyes.

Vincent found that the overall rate of noncompliance (i.e., not using the drops sufficiently as judged by the physician) was 58%. In itself, this high rate is not surprising and is consistent with noncompliance rates for the treatment of many other problems. Knowledge about the positive effects of the drops was a significant factor in compliance. Fifty-five percent of those who were knowledgeable about the drops complied adequately, while only 26% of those who were not sufficiently knowledgeable complied. What is most disturbing, however, is that 45% of those who knew about the therapeutic effects of the drops were still noncompliant!

Some of the sample had already lost vision in one eye due to glaucoma. This is an especially interesting group since they can still see adequately with one eye, but are almost certainly aware that unless they check the course of the glaucoma they will lose vision entirely in both eyes. Did this feedback increase compliance? Yes, but only by 18%. The compliance rate was 59% for those who were not yet blind in either eye, while those who were blind in one eye showed a 41% noncompliance rate. What is striking is that 41% of those with glaucoma who knew that the drops would help and who were legally blind in one eye continued to be noncompliant. This example is dramatic only because glaucoma is a problem that is not complicated by personality factors or by serious side effects of treatment that would interfere with patients' compliance.

The glaucoma example is not any more dramatic than the fact that so many people still continue to smoke despite knowing that smoking very substantially increases the risk of disease and death. Nor is it any more dramatic than the number of people with high blood pressure who do not exercise or control their diets and the many people with other illnesses who are aware of the risks of noncompliance but continue to behave in ways that threaten their health.

There is one factor that seems to be involved in ambivalence about adhering to medical regimens that we have not seen discussed in the literature, but which we have observed in ourselves and others: people may not comply because to do so would be an unpleasant reminder of their weakened state of health, and the reminder can be avoided by noncompliance. Adherence behaviors like going to the doctor, taking a pill, and reading one's blood sugar are all reminders that we have a health problem. That reminder might create negative affect that we avoid, at least in the short run, by acting as if we don't have a problem.

This phenomenon was experienced by one of us (DEE). He was diagnosed with a serious, life-threatening condition. Shortly after the diagnosis, he was given a considerable amount of printed material about the nature of the disease and treatment options. All of his life he had sought out all the information he could find before making an important decision. In this case, however, he put the information into a folder without reading it. Every time he opened the folder and started to read the material in it, he began to feel agitated rather than calmed by the information. He would begin to create catastrophic pictures in his head and then, to relieve his anxiety, he placed the material back in the folder.

There was a part of him that wanted to digest the information, take charge of his medical care, and make informed decisions. There was also another part of him that became frightened and felt out of control, and sought to avoid any reminders of his health problems in order to reduce his anxiety. It took some time before he was able to absorb the information and become an active participant in his medical treatment.

BEHAVIORS REFLECTING RESISTANCE AND NONADHERENCE IN HEALTH CARE

Most experts in the health field (Dimatteo & DiNicola, 1982) agree that nonadherence to medical regimens is multidimensional, involving variables relating to the patient, the physician, the relationship between the patient and the physician, the illness, and whether treatment is preventive or remedial. Meichenbaum and Turk (1987) have described a variety of behaviors that characterize adherence. See Table 1.2.

Despite the differences between psychotherapy and medical health care, the phenomena of resistance and ambivalence are very prevalent in both areas. If we can help people resolve their ambivalence and reduce their resistance to treatment, we can dramatically increase success rates in both areas.

TABLE 1.2. Behaviors Associated with Health Care Nonadherence

---

1. Not entering into or discontinuing a treatment program.
2. Missing referral and follow-up appointments.
3. Not taking prescribed medications as directed.
4. Not following recommended lifestyle changes (e.g., regarding stress, diet, or exercise) at all or sufficiently.
5. Not carrying out home-based therapeutic regimens or doing so less often than recommended.
6. Engaging in health risk behaviors (e.g., smoking, alcohol abuse, or drug abuse).

Note. Adapted from Meichenbaum and Turk (1987). Copyright 1987 by Plenum Press. Adapted by permission.

RESISTANCE AND AMBIVALENCE
IN SELF-DIRECTED CHANGE

We need not go to the literature on health compliance for examples of resistant ambivalence. Every day, we encounter people (including ourselves) who are trying to make lifestyle changes relating to such problems as overeating, smoking, drinking, diet, exercise, stress reduction, and procrastination, and not succeeding despite the fact that there are potentially effective strategies available. For example, there are numerous diets and programs available (e.g., Weight Watchers) which, if followed, would guarantee significant weight loss. The challenge is not to come up with yet another diet or program, but to solve the problem of noncompliance with effective programs that already exist.

I (HA) regularly conduct informal surveys of students in my undergraduate and graduate classes regarding self-change efforts by asking them to respond to the following question: "How many of your are currently trying to make some personal changes that you believe would improve the quality of your life?" The vast majority of students raise their hands. I then follow up with the question "How many of you consider your self-change efforts unsuccessful?" Once again, the majority raise their hands.

Some of the most common self-change attempts involve weight loss; dietary changes (e.g., switching to low-carbohydrate diets); increasing exercise; reducing stress; reducing or eliminating cigarette, alcohol, or drug use; getting more organized; working more or working less; and meeting deadlines. Others are more relationship-based and include becoming more assertive and expressive of one's needs; controlling one's temper; communicating better; becoming more aware of one's feelings; being more attentive to one's partner; becoming less dependent on one's partner; and spending more time with family and friends.

What we see in struggles with self-change is consistent with our definition of ambivalence. Repeated cycles of attempts and failures, partial successes, and outright failure are more the rule than the exception. To make matters worse, a very high percentage of those who succeed initially are unable to maintain the change over time (Brownell et al., 1986).

In an interesting study of New Year's resolutions in college students, Marlatt and Kaplan (1972) found that the most common one was to lose weight, with 38% of the sample resolving to lose weight. Other categories of resolutions included smoking, physical health, relationships, academic conduct, personal traits and dispositions, and personal behavior. Most subjects listed several resolutions. Marlatt followed his subjects for a 3-month period and found that the majority of them had not lost any weight during this time. In other areas of resolution to change, Marlatt found that 62% of the women reported breaking at least one resolution during the 3 months, while 50% of the men did so. The phenomena of resistance and ambivalence are apparent not only in the context of treatment with a health care professional, but within ourselves and our attempts to change for the better.

SUMMARY

Despite the importance of the construct of resistance in psychotherapy, health care, and self-change, we know relatively little about it. There has been very little empirical work on the subject. The literature consists mostly of thoughts and observations from clinicians of different theoretical persuasions. Theories of psychotherapy provide different definitions of resistance and different ways of thinking about it. This situation has led to a fragmentation of knowledge that has impeded progress toward better research and practice in the area. In this book, we present an integrative framework for understanding and working with resistant ambivalence that draws from different theoretical points of view. Instead of asking "Why do people resist?", we ask "Why don't people change?" Our goals in this book are to provide ways of understanding and working with resistant ambivalence to help people remove obstacles to personal change.

CHAPTER 2

Theories of Resistance and Ambivalence

In this chapter, we review how different kinds of psychotherapy deal with resistance. We consider the four major approaches to psychotherapy—psychoanalytic, cognitive-behavioral, humanistic-experiential, and family systems—as well as some of the major variations within each. We also review several more recent proposals for understanding resistance that do not clearly fit into any of the four major schools of psychotherapy. In the review that follows, we consider how each addresses four questions:

1. What changes are resisted?
2. What behaviors define the presence of resistance?
3. Why is resistance occurring?
4. How do those therapies work with resistance in clinical practice?

PSYCHOANALYTIC PERSPECTIVES ON RESISTANCE

Resistance plays a central role in some psychoanalytic theories and little or no role in others. This review focuses on views that are currently influential in psychoanalytic theory and practice. These include Freudian, object relations, attachment, and relational theories.

The concept of resistance is central to Freudian psychoanalytic approaches and, to a lesser extent, to more modern versions of psycho-analytic thinking.[1] In the Freudian psychoanalytic perspective, the question "Why do people resist?" becomes "Why don't people change symptoms and repetitive maladaptive interpersonal patterns, both of which persist despite the distress that they create?" In this view, instinctual drives, usually representing sexual or aggressive motivations, press for gratification. Since these drives pose problems for the ego and are unacceptable to the superego, they undergo repression. As Eagle (1999) points out, neurotic symptoms and patterns of behavior are attempts to resolve a dilemma:

> To fail to gratify instinctual wishes entails the danger of being over-whelmed by excessive excitation, and to attempt to gratify instinctual wishes openly (that is, fail to repress them) risks intense anxiety which also entails the danger of being overwhelmed by excitation. However distress-ing neurotic symptoms and neurotic patterns may be, they are deemed, at some level, as preferable to the dangers entailed in the available alterna-tives. Thus, in Freudian theory, resistance to change occurs because the symptoms or patterns of behavior to be changed are serving the vital functions of permitting partial gratification and, at the same time, avoiding intense anxiety. (p. 8)

As long as these wishes remain unconscious, they cannot be grati-fied in reality nor can the person learn to live a satisfying life without their fulfillment. Change cannot occur until these wishes become con-scious. Because of the operation of the pleasure principle, any attempts to make them conscious or to change them will raise anxiety that will in turn result in resistant avoidance. Resistance, then, is seen as a predictable and inevitable part of the change process. In fact, the occurrence of resistance in psychoanalytic therapy signals that the work is getting closer to the core conflicts underlying the neurotic symptoms.

Freud (1926/1959) described five varieties of resistance. These are presented in Table 2.1.

In the Freudian view, there is a core conflict between id wishes and impulses that seek expression and the superego that seeks to prevent their expression. The pressure of the id wishes causes anxiety, which the defenses seek to reduce. Neurotic symptoms in general and repetitive

---

[1]Eagle (1999) has done a masterful job of extracting the essences of these perspectives on re-sistance, and this section draws from Eagle's seminal work.

TABLE 2.1. Types of Resistance in Freudian Psychoanalytic Theory

1. *Repression*: Keeping painful thoughts, fantasies, wishes, and feelings from conscious awareness in order to defend against anxiety. Since repression is the basis for the defenses of the ego, the operation of any defenses like denial, projection, and reaction formation constitute examples of resistance.

2. *The repetition compulsion*: The unconscious tendency to repeat in adult relationships patterns of behavior relevant to seeking satisfaction of childhood wishes and object choices.

3. *Transference*: The manifestation of the repetition compulsion in the relationship with the therapist. For example, a patient whose interpersonal relationships throughout his or her life have been characterized by dependency will also try to form a dependent relationship with the therapist.

4. *Secondary gain*: The person receives some benefits from the symptom (e.g., greater attention from spouse).

5. *Superego resistance of a sense of guilt and a need for punishment:* This proposal of Freud's has received relatively little attention in the subsequent psychoanalytic literature and is not discussed further here.

maladaptive interpersonal patterns in and out of therapy constitute a "compromise formation," or a partial solution to the conflict. The symptoms, or the maladaptive repetitive interpersonal patterns, then, are solutions to a problem of anxiety. *At the most general level, Freudian psychoanalytic theory proposes that resistant behaviors occur in order to reduce the anxiety associated with the awareness of the unconscious conflicts and particularly of the drives or wishes that form their basis.* As Eagle (1999) points out, resistance is not to change per se, but to experiencing painful feelings.

In secondary gain, the person receives some benefits from the symptom, as may be true in the case of a depressed woman who feels unloved by her partner and whose depression leads to greater attention and concern from him. Change may threaten an important relationship that has accommodated to the symptoms, as in the case of a man with agoraphobia whose symptoms draw his wife close to him. The man may believe that eliminating the symptoms will distance his wife from him, and resist change as a result.

Other Freudian psychoanalytic writers have elaborated on these themes (cf. Basch, 1982; Blatt & Ehrlich, 1982; Dewald, 1982; Messer,

2002; Schlesinger, 1982). For example, Blatt and Ehrlich (1982) suggest that resistance is a way to maintain the familiar and predictable status quo even though it is associated with distress.

Westen (personal communication, 2003) has suggested that the client both seeks change and fears it because change means not only doing and perhaps feeling the unfamiliar, but also involves undoing ways of thinking and behaving that help regulate affect but ultimately cause more pain than they are preventing. He further suggested that

> in many respects, psychodynamic treatment is as much about de-automatizing the automatized as it is about making the unconscious conscious, expanding the patient's capacity for new kinds of relatedness, or altering ways of viewing the self (three of the most prominent views of therapeutic change in psychoanalysis today). This paradox—the promise that if the patient gives up familiar ways of thinking and protecting him/herself from unpleasant emotions s/he might end up feeling better in the long run—is the source of resistance in dynamic treatments.

There are a variety of modern post-Freudian psychoanalytic views of resistance, including control–mastery theory (Weiss, Sampson, & the Mount Zion Psychotherapy Group, 1986) and attachment and object relations theories (e.g., Bowlby, 1969, 1973; Fairbairn, 1952; Mitchell, 1988; Stern, 1985). In these views, the general question of "Why do people resist change?" is transformed into the specific question "Why do people resist changing relationship patterns that bring them distress?" While these theories may differ on the nature of the danger, they all agree that resistance is a response to perceived danger and the anxiety that accompanies it.

Control–mastery theory is based on the importance of "unconscious pathogenic beliefs" that are acquired early in life and lead to neurotic behavior and distress. Weiss, Sampson, and the Mount Zion Psychotherapy Group (1986) propose that symptoms and maladaptive interpersonal patterns are attempts at mastery, that is, efforts to disconfirm these beliefs. The beliefs are difficult to modify because they are unconscious, and possibly, as Eagle (1999) suggests, because of the fear that if they are put to the test, they will be confirmed. Eagle (1999) gives the example of a man whose pathogenic beliefs include the idea that separating from his parents will destroy him. The man can avoid the anxiety and guilt associated with this belief by failing to become independent of his parents.

Attachment and object relations theories (Bowlby, 1969, 1973; Fairbairn, 1952; Mitchell, 1988; Stern, 1985) suggest that infants develop internal mental representations of their caregivers and their interactions with them. These representations are considered to be relatively stable and resistant to change. They influence our perceptions of and expectations regarding new relationships, so that we tend to perceive and structure new relationships in ways that are consistent with our early mental representations.

Attachment theories also suggest another reason for resistance to change: repetitive maladaptive interpersonal patterns are maintained because they provide some degree of security in fulfilling one's attachment needs. Relinquishing these attachment patterns causes anxiety triggered by a sense of betrayal of the attachment figures, leaving the person in an empty psychological world, thereby threatening his or her identity. Thus, repeating old patterns brings some degree of security, while changing them leads to insecurity that will manifest itself as anxiety about change.

Carrying forward old patterns from the past is a key part of the picture. Another is what Wachtel (1982) has aptly called "vicious cycles," that is, that unresolved conflicts from the past cause us to structure our present in a manner that confirms the old patterns. Our perceptions, colored by our past history, lead us to perceive new situations as similar to old ones, eliciting and confirming the old repetitive interpersonal patterns. As a result, we elicit behaviors from others that are congruent with our early mental representations. In this way, our old patterns are continually reinforced by our present encounters. For example, a man whose internal representations are that female caretakers cannot be trusted to provide nurturance may act in an aloof and suspicious manner with women, leading them to respond with cautious distance, thereby fulfilling his expectation that they won't nurture him.

Wachtel (1993) has also suggested that every therapist communication carries two messages: a focal message that is the overt content (e.g., the therapist communicating his or her understanding of the client or his or her dynamics) and a "meta-message" that conveys an attitude about what is being conveyed in the focal message. He suggests that it is the meta-message, as read by the client, that is often responsible for resistance and therapeutic failure. For example, a therapist can communicate that the client spends a great deal of life trying to please others in a way that will more likely be perceived as supportive or in a way that will more likely be perceived as critical. In general, Wachtel argues that there are facilitative and nonfacilitative ways to say things in therapy. He writes:

> A key to conducting an inquiry in a way that does not create needless resistance . . . is to keep clearly in mind that the patient is most often in conflict. Often, the primary challenge facing the therapist is to find a route into the experience of conflict, to access the complexity beneath the apparently monolithic attitudes that (at a terribly high cost) protect the patient from the less acknowledged side of his conflict. Finding potential tiny chinks in the defensive armor without becoming adversarial is the key to inquiry that is effective and therapeutic. (1993, p. 89)

Wachtel also points to the dialectic between acceptance and change, emphasizing the need for the therapist to be able to see the world through the client's eyes, understanding and appreciating his or her perspective and why the client has found it necessary to live his or her life as he or she does. On the other hand, the therapist must keep in mind that the client has sought therapy because something is wrong and that the therapist is an agent of change. He suggests that if the therapist emphasizes one of these poles at the expense of the other, change is unlikely to occur. Understanding that the client is in conflict helps the therapist to respond effectively to the client's wanting to stay the same and wanting to change. Thus, Wachtel emphasizes the importance of conflict in resistance.

Bromberg (1998), an interpersonal-relational psychoanalyst, describes a shift in psychoanalytic thinking away from a view of resistance as motivated by repression and avoidance. He suggests that many psychoanalytic writers have been moving toward a view of the self as a configuration of different states of consciousness engaging in an ongoing dialectic while maintaining a healthy illusion of unitary selfhood. According to Bromberg, this view originated with Breuer and Freud and has continued to influence psychoanalytic thinking through the writings of such authors as Balint (1968), Laing (1969), Searles (1977), Sullivan (1947, 1953), and Winnicott (1958, 1971). In Bromberg's view, an understanding of dissociation and trauma can provide greater insight into mental life and resistance than an understanding of repression and avoidance. Dissociative processes create these different self-states that occur in both health and pathology. Each self-state is engaged in internal negotiation with the realities, values, affects, and perspectives of the others. Bromberg (1998) writes that "resistance can be usefully reframed as part of an enacted dialectical process of meaning construction, rather than an archaeological barrier preventing the surfacing of disavowed reality" (p. 206). He suggests that there is a dialectic between opposing parts of the self, and that resistance can be seen as a result of this dialectic between stability and change. While change is desirable and sought, it also means losing something old, a loss that is frightening and therefore resisted. He suggests that change is resisted because we need to protect our sense of a stable and unitary self.

Although Bromberg's views are couched in the language of psychoanalysis, they are very close to the humanistic-experiential perspective, the work of Stiles (1997), and the position taken in this book, all of which are discussed in this chapter and the next.

What Changes Are Resisted?

1. Awareness of unconscious wishes and drives which that cause anxiety.
2. Changing repetitive and maladaptive interpersonal patterns.
3. Changing pathogenic beliefs and internal object relations.

What Behaviors Define the Presence of Resistance?

Freudian psychoanalysis focuses primarily on those *behaviors that attempt to avoid painful awareness or insights.* Behaviors that are considered to be manifestations of ego mechanisms of defense (e.g., repression, denial, projection) constitute resistant behaviors.

In addition, Freudian and other related views also emphasize that continued engagement in long-term repetitive and maladaptive interpersonal patterns indicate resistance.

In psychoanalytic therapy, the therapist must rely on a considerable amount of inference to judge behaviors as resistant, since he or she cannot usually make this judgment on the face value of the behavior. For example, consider the case of a man who says to his therapist, "No, my wife doesn't make me angry when she's critical of me. I feel that way about her sometimes too." If we focus only on the overt content of this statement, we may conclude that it simply reflects the man's accurate report that his wife's criticism does not make him angry, and not reflect resistance. By contrast, if prior therapeutic work with him had revealed his tendency to deny angry feelings because they make him anxious, then we may consider the same statement as reflecting the operation of repression or denial, and therefore indicative of resistance.

In summary, behaviors that reflect resistance in psychoanalytic therapies are:

1. Overt or covert behaviors that attempt to avoid painful awareness or insights. Often these are ego mechanisms of defense (e.g., repression, denial, projection).
2. Ongoing engagement in long-term repetitive interpersonal patterns despite the fact that they continue to cause distress and lack of gratification.

Why Is Resistance Occurring?

1. Anxiety reduction through avoidance of anxiety-generating insight into or awareness of one's unconscious drives and impulses.
2. "Diablos conocidos" (familiar devils): The security and predictability of the familiar.
3. Protection of a sense of stable identity by not changing.
4. Fear of change.
5. Unconscious pathogenic beliefs that maintain symptomatic behaviors.
6. Vicious cycles in which the person's internal object representations from early in life are confirmed by the way the person perceives and structures his or her world in the present.
7. Secondary gain in which the person receives benefit from the symptomatic behavior.

How Do Psychoanalytic Approaches Work with Resistance in Clinical Practice?

There are many variations of psychoanalytic therapies. This section focuses on Freudian psychoanalytic therapy and how it works with resistance, since it is basic to all other psychoanalytic approaches. Strupp and Binder (1984), writing from a Freudian perspective, suggest that resistance is not just an obstacle to change and a problem to overcome, but is at the very heart of how change occurs in psychoanalysis and psychoanalytic psychotherapy. Resistance is expected and occurs in the transference relationship, in which much of the work of psychoanalytic therapy occurs. In the course of the relationship with the therapist, the client will manifest resistances in the form of defense mechanisms (e.g., repression, denial, reaction formation) and will enact in the therapy relationship the various repetitive maladaptive interpersonal patterns of behavior that parallel his or her interpersonal problems outside of therapy. The therapist's main strategy is interpretation of the client's emotional experience, linking the present enactments in the transference relationship to conflicting earlier experiences. Interpretation is directed at insight in which the client becomes able to connect his or her current experience in the transference to those older conflicts, and comes to understand how his or her present behavior is a manifestation of these unresolved conflicts. This learning is thought to be effective because it is based in experience in the transference, and not just on discussions of early history.

Alexander and French's (1946) concept of the "corrective emotional experience" was out of favor in psychoanalytic circles for many years, but is now increasingly accepted among modern psychoanalytic therapists. Alexander and French suggested that change occurs when the client relives chronic conflictual patterns of behavior and experiences in the transference relationship, *and experiences a different outcome in the relationship with the therapist.* For example, a man who had a very critical father and subsequently experienced authority figures as critical might try to provoke the analytic therapist into critical reactions without consciously realizing that he is doing so. When the psychoanalytic therapist does not respond as the patient expects, the client can begin to reevaluate the view of authority figures that he has carried forward from the past, and begin to change this view.

In a brief summary, a Freudian analytic therapist works with resistance in the following ways:

1. Therapist interpretations identify defensive avoidance/repetitive interpersonal patterns in and out of therapy.
2. The therapist's interpretations link defensive avoidance/repetitive interpersonal enactments in the transference relationship to the client's early conflictual experiences.
3. The client's insight that the present defensive avoidance/interpersonal patterns are manifestations of earlier conflicts reduces the client's need to engage in these patterns.
4. The client undergoes a corrective emotional experience. When the psychoanalytic therapist does not respond to the enactments as the client expected, the client begins to question the need to engage in them and begins to change them.

COGNITIVE-BEHAVIORAL THEORIES
OF RESISTANCE

Kendall, Krain, and Henin (2000) suggest that cognitive-behavioral therapy (CBT) assumes the interrelatedness of cognitive, emotional, and behavioral variables so that changing one leads to changes in the others. CBT strategies may focus on changing cognition, emotion, or behavior. The masthead of the main CBT journal, *Behavior Therapy*, describes its domain as "the application of behavioral and cognitive sciences to clinical problems."

There are many approaches that constitute CBT (Dobson & Shaw, 1995). Behavior therapy is the historical antecedent of both CBT and cognitive therapy, and still constitutes an important current area of interest in CBT. It emphasizes changes in behavior and emotion, with minimal emphasis on cognition. One of the main behavior therapy approaches is functional analysis, which is based on the work of B. F. Skinner (e.g., 1938, 1953, 1961) and illustrated by the work of Patterson and his associates (e.g., Patterson & Chamberlain, 1994) discussed below. Cognitive therapy emerged as a major direction in the 1970s and includes the work of Beck and his associates (e.g., Beck, Rush, Shaw, & Emery, 1979), and the earlier work of Albert Ellis and his rational-emotive therapy (Ellis, 1962). From the late 1980s to the present, the broader field of CBT has emerged and now encompasses a variety of approaches including behavioral, cognitive, and newer cognitive-behavioral ones as well (e.g., Barlow, 2002).

In order to learn more about CBT views of resistance and noncompliance, we searched for these terms in the indices of several major books in the area (Beck, 1995; Beck et al., 1979; Patterson, 2002; Salkovskis, 1996). These included the classic Beck et al. (1979) work on cognitive therapy for depression, as well as a recent handbook on CBT that included 25 chapters written by leading figures in the field (Patterson, 2002). Neither term appeared in the index of any of these books, suggesting that resistance and noncompliance are not considered to be of major importance in CBT.

Some CBT therapists prefer not to use the term "resistance" at all. For example, Lazarus and Fay (1982) state that "the concept of 'resistance' is probably the most elaborate rationalization that therapists employ to explain their treatment failures" (p. 115). These authors suggest that "by labeling such behaviors as resistance and attributing their causes to this hypothetical state, we avoid searching for the real reasons behind these behaviors" (p. 115). Such CBT therapists may not deny that clients engage in behaviors that interfere with the progress of therapy, but object to calling it resistance.

When CBT therapists do discuss behaviors that interfere with therapy, they are more likely to refer to "noncompliance" with the procedures of CBT, especially homework, than to resistance. For example, Davis and Hollon (1999) suggest that the problems of noncompliance and resistance can be reframed in terms of the question "Why don't cognitive therapy patients always do what we ask them to do?" (p. 34).

Behavioral Approaches to Resistance

The behavioral view of resistance is largely based on a Skinnerian (1938, 1953, 1961) functional-analytic perspective. Functional analysis is aimed at discovering relationships among behaviors, antecedents, consequences, and other classes of events hypothesized to be relevant to the target behaviors. In the behavioral approach, resistance may be due to the use of inappropriate reinforcers, inadequate reinforcement contingencies for the desired behaviors, reinforcement of behaviors that conflict with the goals of therapy, or setting standards for changed performance too high (Leahy, 2001).

Gerald Patterson and his associates (e.g., Chamberlain, Patterson, Reid, Kavanagh, & Forgatch, 1984; Patterson & Chamberlain, 1994; Patterson & Forgatch, 1985) have employed a novel behavioral approach to understanding and studying resistance. Patterson and Chamberlin (1994) suggested that no one theory of resistance can deal adequately with different people and problems. Therefore theories need to be population-specific. Consistent with this view, their model of resistance was developed in their work with the families of antisocial boys and is specific to this population.

Chamberlain et al. (1984) developed a behavioral coding system for resistant behavior for use during parent-training therapy for parents of antisocial boys. They coded three types of resistant behavior: verbalizations reflecting "I can't, verbalizations" reflecting "I won't," and homework completion. Parental resistance was associated with increased teaching and confrontation by the therapist, a greater number of sessions required for treatment, and a reduction in the therapist's liking for the client. Patterson and Forgatch (1985) found that directive behaviors by the therapist were more likely to elicit resistant behaviors in clients, and that supportive behaviors by the therapist were more likely to elicit cooperative behaviors in clients. Patterson and Chamberlain (1994), using an expanded version of the coding system, also examined other variables that might be related to parental resistance including a history of defeats during discipline confrontations with the child; parents' characteristics such as depression or antisocial; stress and social disadvantage; and the skill and intensity of the therapists' attempts to teach and confront the parents during the session.

The approach of Patterson and his associates is noteworthy as much for its theory of resistance in families of antisocial boys as it is for the method of model building. Most theories of resistance can be described as "top-down": they start with broad theoretical constructs and use these to predict and understand resistant behavior in therapy. Patterson takes more of a "bottom-up" approach: he defines potentially interesting classes of behavior and events that might influence their occurrence, and then builds a network of empirically derived relationships that can form a solid basis for theory.

Cognitive Therapy Approaches to Resistance

The basic premise of all cognitive approaches is that our thoughts and interpretations about events largely determine how we react emotionally and behaviorally. In this view, cognition is primary. If we *believe* that a situation is dangerous, we will experience autonomic arousal and tend to avoid it, regardless of whether the situation is truly dangerous or not. *The essence of the cognitive approach is that noncompliant behaviors are based largely on faulty beliefs, assumptions, and schemas.*

Beck's Cognitive Therapy Approach

While Beck et al. (1979) do not specifically discuss "resistance" or "noncompliance," they do address what they call "countertherapeutic beliefs." An example of such a belief is "I know I look at things in a negative way, but I can't change my personality." In cognitive therapy, these beliefs are treated like any other dysfunctional beliefs and identified, examined, and challenged according to the evidence of the person's life.

Beck, Freeman, and Associates (1990) present a fuller discussion of resistance in cognitive therapy in the context of their discussion of personality disorders. They prefer to use the term "noncollaboration" to avoid the pejorative implications that they see in terms like "resistance" or "noncompliance." They discuss a number of reasons that problems in collaboration may occur (see Table 2.2). While many of these center on a client's dysfunctional beliefs, some address therapist and environmental factors that may cause noncooperation.

Beck et al. (1990) and other theorists who have developed more recent cognitive formulations (e.g., Young, Klosko, & Weishaar, 2003) have gone beyond thoughts, beliefs, and attitudes to suggest that psychological problems are caused by cognitive structures called "schemas" that cause distorted thoughts and images in specific situations (Dobson & Shaw, 1995). These schemas are thought to be shaped by experience, to

TABLE 2.2. Reasons for Problems in Collaboration Therapy

- The patient may lack the skills to be collaborative.
- The therapist may lack the skill to develop collaboration.
- Environmental stressors may preclude change or reinforce dysfunctional behavior.
- Patients' ideas and beliefs regarding their potential failure in therapy.
- Patients' ideas and beliefs regarding effects of their changing on others.
- Patients' fears regarding changing and the "new self."
- The patient's and therapist's dysfunctional beliefs may be harmoniously blended.
- Poor socialization to the treatment model.
- Secondary gain from maintaining the dysfunctional pattern.
- Poor timing of interventions.
- Lacks in patient motivation.
- Patients' rigidity may foil compliance.
- Poor impulse control.
- Unrealistic therapy goals.
- Unstated therapy goals.
- Vague and amorphous therapy goals.
- Lack of agreement between patient and therapist regarding therapy goals.
- Frustration about lack of progress on the part of therapist or patient.
- Patients' perceptions of lowered status or self-esteem attributed to becoming a patient.

Note. From Beck, Freeman, and Associates (1990). Copyright 1990 by The Guilford Press. Reprinted by permission.

reside in long-term memory, and to affect a number of cognitive processes like attention, information processing, encoding, and recall. Schemas may be available to awareness or they may operate outside of awareness. Recent views of schemas have emphasized that they are not just cognitive structures, but also have emotional components and action tendencies (Barlow, 2002). Emotions consistent with a schema elicit cognitions congruent with that schema and vice versa. Schemas may be latent and activated by certain life events. For example, a therapist who suggests a homework assignment to a client to be more assertive with others may activate a schema about abandonment that could interfere with the client carrying out the assignment.

Beck et al. (1990) describe schemas as vulnerabilities that may be activated by certain life events. They are established early in childhood and lead to selective attention and recall of information consistent with the schema. For example, a dependent person would selectively attend to and remember information consistent with his or her schema that he or she must have the attention and support of others to survive adequately in the world. They suggest that avoidance and compensation are two coping styles people adopt to deal with these schemas. *Avoidance* is the tendency to stay away or to escape from situations in which the schemas might be activated. As an example, the depressed person may avoid or try to escape from situations that require autonomy and independent functioning since these situations activate his or her schema for dependency. By contrast, *compensation* is the tendency to avoid the distress caused by activation of the schema by engaging in excessive levels of behavior to gain the acceptance and approval of others. These styles lead to resistance in therapy when the therapist tries to address these schemas therapeutically and the client reacts by avoidance or compensation to keep from examining the schema.

The cognitive model of psychopathology hypothesizes that different disorders are associated with different cognitive schemas that serve as vulnerability factors for the negative thinking in specific situations. For example, many depressed persons have self-schemas like "I'm defective" or "I'm inadequate," while the self-schemas of anxious people relate to vulnerability and danger. While people can be aware of the thoughts that reflect these schemas, the schemas themselves are hypothesized to usually operate outside of conscious awareness. In this context, there are schemas that relate to resistance or noncompliance. Leahy (2001) has presented a thorough discussion of these; we review his work shortly.

Albert Ellis's Rational-Emotive Behavior Therapy Approach

Ellis's well-known rational-emotive behavior therapy (REBT) predated the cognitive therapy of Beck and others (e.g., Ellis, 1958, 1962). Consistent with a cognitive model, Ellis proposed that beliefs mediate between events, on the one hand, and feelings and behaviors, on the other. One factor that distinguishes Ellis's REBT from Beck's cognitive therapy and other cognitive therapy approaches is the postulation of specific irrational beliefs that underlie dysfunctional emotions and behaviors including resistance. Ellis (2002) proposes three basic beliefs that cause emotional distress and resistance:

1. "It shouldn't be so hard for me to change, so I'll give up trying."
2. "If I tried to change and failed, it would prove what an inadequate person I am."
3. "People close to me should realize how hard it is for me to change and should be more helpful, and if they don't, I'm not going to bother to change."

In his book on resistance, Ellis (2002) also presents a comprehensive discussion of different reasons why resistance may occur. These are presented in Table 2.3.

TABLE 2.3. Reasons for Resistance in Rational-Emotive Behavior Therapy

- Severe emotional disturbance.
- Extremely low frustration tolerance.
- Fear of disclosure and shame.
- Feelings of hopelessness.
- Self-punishment.
- Pessimism, depressive outlook, and lack of risk taking.
- Perfection and grandiosity.
- Fear of change.
- Reactance/rebelliousness.
- Client's hidden agendas.
- Unusual biological and neurological conditions.
- Resistance due to problems in the therapeutic relationship.

Ellis proposes that therapists work with resistance as they do with any other problem in psychotherapy: by identifying and challenging the underlying irrational beliefs, and by confronting the client with the fact that he or she must change these beliefs if he or she wishes to change his or her feelings and behaviors.

Cognitive-Behavioral Therapy Approaches

The view of noncompliance as a reflection of underlying dysfunctional and distorted thinking has been elaborated and modified by many others including Davis and Hollon (1999), Goldfried and Davison (1976), Leahy (2002), Meichenbaum and Gilmore (1982), and Newman (2002). These authors elaborate on models that are basically cognitive but also include significant behavioral elements.

Goldfried and Davison (1976) wrote that "any difficulties occurring during the course of therapy should more appropriately be traced to the therapist's inadequate or incomplete evaluation of the case" (p. 17). Goldfried (1982) suggested that noncompliance may reflect any one or more of the following: "a direct sampling of the client's presenting problem itself; the client's other problems; pessimism about changing; fear of changing; minimal motivation to change; psychological reactance; overburdening the client with too many homework assignments and interfering contingencies in the client's environment" (pp. 104–105).

Davis and Hollon (1999) suggest that in addition to faulty beliefs, factors external to the client might create resistance, including therapist factors and insufficiency of the model. These may include the therapist's negative expectations about change in the client; failure on the part of the therapist to correctly conceptualize what the patient needs and what needs to be done; an overly routinized and rigid approach on the part of the therapist that does not adequately adapt the treatment to the particular client and his or her problems; and therapist imposition of attitudes or values on the client in a dogmatic fashion. Meichenbaum and Turk (1987) have provided a comprehensive account of "treatment adherence," a term they prefer to "compliance" because they believe that adherence connotes more active, voluntary, mutual, and cooperative involvement in the treatment program than the term "noncompliance," which emphasizes clients' more passive cooperation with the advice and suggestions of the health care professional. They discuss client beliefs as mediators of nonadherence, and point to the importance of the client's beliefs that he or she has the ability to carry out the treatment program and that carrying out the treatment will make a difference. In addition, these authors discuss a number of other interrelated factors that contribute to nonadherence. These include:

1. The quality of the relationship between the client and the health care provider.
2. The importance of good client education that includes the nature of the expectations of the client and the health care provider about their respective roles and responsibilities in the treatment.
3. The need for a treatment regimen that is not too demanding for the client.
4. The need for the client to have the necessary skills or resources to carry out the treatment.

Robert Leahy, a cognitive-behavioral therapist, proposed what he calls an "integrative social-cognitive model of resistance" (Leahy, 2001, p. 20). Consistent with a cognitive-behavioral view, Leahy sees resistance primarily as noncompliance and asserts that resistance refers to "how a patient does not comply with a specific role defined by the therapist" (p. 21).

While firmly based in CBT, Leahy's is an integrated approach, drawing selectively from psychoanalytic, behavioral, and cognitive therapy, as well as from economic theory and basic research in psychology on emotion, cognition, and social behavior. He suggests that each dimension of resistance represents "a relatively self-contained style of thinking" that "needs to be understood and addressed in therapy within its own rules and logic" (p. 21). The dimensions discussed by Leahy include:

- *Validation resistance.* This is "the demand for understanding, empathy, and care from the therapist—often to the exclusion of problem solving or a rational perspective" (2001, p. 58). When such demands are not satisfactorily met, the patient may resort to a number of strategies that are resistant including rumination, escalation of intensity, devaluation of the therapist, emotional distancing, splitting the transference, and noncompliance with homework.
- *Self-consistency.* Some instances of resistance are caused by the tendency of people to maintain self-consistency, predictability, and control

that is associated with their negative thinking. In this context, giving up the negative thinking will lead to uncomfortable states that are avoided by maintaining the current state of affairs.

• *Schematic resistance.* Leahy suggests that schemas are self-perpetuating and maintain themselves through selective attention and memory to information that is consistent with the schema and avoidance or devaluing of information that challenges it. As a result, attempts to try to change maladaptive schemas will meet with resistance.

• *Moral resistance.* People will resist change when they perceive that the therapist is challenging their basic moral or ethical beliefs (i.e., their "shoulds"). They will cling to such beliefs even though they may cause distress. Therapist arguments based on rationality and utility will be futile in attempts to modify them. For example, belief in a "just world" in which bad things happen to bad people may be used as justification for the patient's pain and distress. Attempts to alleviate the distress by challenging this very basic moral belief will be resisted.

• *Victim resistance.* This is resistance caused by the client's view that his or her misfortunes are the fault of others. Such persons require validation and acknowledgment of their own innocence and others' guilt. When they perceive that the therapist is not providing such validation, resistance may result.

• *Risk aversion.* Leahy suggests that one aspect of resistance seen particularly in depressed persons is that they typically see the risks of change as involving a greater likelihood of negativity and loss than of positivity and gain. Because of this, they are resistant to attempting change.

• *Self-handicapping.* In this category, clients engage in a variety of strategies that involve self-handicapping and negative self-verification for self-protective reasons. For example, a person may avoid evaluating him- or herself under optimal circumstances in order to avoid the potential distress that may arise from finding out that he or she does not live up to his or her own standards.

Finally, in a proposal unusual for a cognitive-behavioral therapist, Leahy discusses how resistance may arise from the therapeutic relationship due to the reactions of the therapist to the client, that is, countertransference. He discusses how the reactions of the therapist to the client and the presence of certain schemas in the therapist that relate to the client can cause resistance.

What Changes Are Resisted?

1. Compliance with the procedures of CBT during the session. Leahy's (2001) description of the tasks of cognitive therapy gives some idea of the specific behaviors that define noncompliance in CBT. He describes these tasks as emphasis on the here and now, structured sessions, continuity across sessions, problem-solving orientation, rational thinking, collaboration with the therapist, psychoeducation and information sharing, an active role for both patient and therapist, accountability as evidenced by identifying and measuring goals and attainment of goals, and compliance with self-help assignments.
2. Compliance with between-session homework assignments or experiments.
3. Perhaps the core changes that are resisted in CBT are *changes in distorted thoughts, attitudes, beliefs, and schemas underlying symptomatic and resistant (noncompliant) behaviors.*

What Behaviors Define the Presence of Resistance?

The core feature of resistant behaviors in CBT is noncompliance with either in-session or between-session procedures. However, any therapy-interfering behavior is considered to be resistance. Newman (1994), writing from a cognitive therapy perspective, described a number of behaviors reflecting resistance. These are presented in Table 2.4.

Why Is Resistance Occurring?

1. The therapist's use of inappropriate reinforcers, inadequate reinforcement contingencies for desired behaviors, reinforcement of behaviors that conflict with the goals of therapy, or setting standards for changed performance too high.
2. The client's faulty beliefs and assumptions and the schemas on which they are based.
3. The therapist's negative attitudes or lack of skill.
4. The therapist's inadequate or incomplete evaluation of the case.
5. Client characteristics such as poor impulse control or rigidity.
6. Problems in the relationship between therapist and client.

TABLE 2.4. Behaviors Reflecting Resistance

1. Refusal or other failure to follow through on therapy homework assignments.
2. Repeatedly making decisions and taking actions that run counter to what was agreed upon in session.
3. High levels of expressed emotion toward the therapist ranging from excessive flirtation to overt hostility.
4. In-session avoidances such as silences, overly frequent usage of "I don't know," and abrupt topic shifts.
5. Gratuitous debates with the therapist.
6. Relapses in functioning that occur when the client has difficulty enduring the increased anxiety that accompanies initial attempts to function more adaptively.
7. Repeated misinterpretations of the therapist's comments.
8. Ill-advised interruptions of therapy or inappropriate scheduling of sessions (e.g., on a crisis basis only).
9. Attempts to prolong therapy unduly.
10. Placing unreasonable demands on the therapist.

Note. Adapted from Newman (1994). Copyright 1994 by John Wiley & Sons. Adapted by permission.

How Do Cognitive-Behavioral Approaches Work with Resistance in Clinical Practice?

From a behavioral point of view, resistant behavior is seen as elicited by certain stimuli and maintained by response consequences. In this view, when a client manifests resistant behaviors, the therapist needs to conduct an analysis of the situation to determine what may be eliciting the resistance (e.g., confronting behaviors; see Patterson & Chamberlain, 1994) and what events in and out of therapy may be reinforcing resistant behavior (e.g., a spouse who pays excessive attention to the client's problematic behavior, inadvertently reinforcing such behavior). *One strategy of working with resistance is to change the eliciting stimuli and reinforcers that maintain such behaviors.*

More cognitively oriented CBT therapists (e.g., Beck et al., 1979; J. S. Beck, 1995; Dobson & Shaw, 1995) work with resistance or noncompliance in exactly the same way that they work with other problems: *by helping clients to correct their dysfunctional thoughts and beliefs and to modify the schemas underlying their resistance and other related problem behaviors.* Cognitive therapists help clients to identify the thoughts and beliefs associated with resistance, examine the evidence for and against these thoughts, and construct new balanced thoughts that better fit the evidence of their lives. Work proceeds from thoughts to beliefs to schemas. In addition to reviewing evidence from the past relating to these thoughts and beliefs, Beck's cognitive therapy emphasizes the construction of *experiments* that clients may try during the week to test out the accuracy of certain thoughts and beliefs that may be related to resistance. For example, a cognitive therapist working with a client who is acting in a noncompliant manner will inquire into the thoughts that are associated with noncompliance. A thought that might cause noncompliance might be "I'll never be able to change." This thought would then be recast as a hypothesis to be examined. The client and the therapist both examine evidence from the person's past in different areas in which he or she has attempted to change. They would likely find some instances where the client has been successfully able to change that might lead to a modification of the negative thought to something like "While change has been difficult, I have been successful at it in some times in the past, and I might be successful if I try to change this problem." This latter belief should be associated with reduced noncompliance. The job of client and therapist would be to unearth as many of the thoughts and beliefs underlying the noncompliance as they can and subject them all to this kind of cognitive analysis. Ellis's REBT (e.g., Ellis, 1994) is also directed at modifying underlying thoughts and beliefs, but does so in a more challenging and confronting manner.

HUMANISTIC-EXPERIENTIAL APPROACHES TO RESISTANCE

Humanistic-experiential approaches include client-centered therapy, gestalt therapy, process-experiential therapy, transpersonal psychology, and several others. Several consistent themes or threads run through these approaches. First, they all assume that people are fundamentally striving to live a good life and to actualize their potential, although they may sometimes act in ways that are destructive or evil. Second, they share an emphasis on the "whole person" that includes body, feelings, and intellect (some approaches also add a transpersonal/spiritual dimension). These approaches suggest that people seek wholeness and integration of the self. Third, they all emphasize change and development. People are abundantly curious and have a need for a wide range of experiences. Humanistic-experiential therapists believe that people will naturally continue to grow if they do not limit themselves and their potential. Fourth, humanistic-experiential approaches are rooted in a fundamental acceptance of clients and their worldviews.

This section focuses on two of the major humanistic-experiential views: Carl Rogers's (e.g., Rogers, 1951, 1961) client-centered therapy and gestalt therapy derived from the work of Fritz Perls and his associates (Perls, Hefferline, & Goodman, 1951; Kepner, 1987; Polster & Polster, 1973).

Client-Centered Therapy

A revealing insight into Carl Rogers's way of thinking about resistance comes from the index to his classic book *Client-Centered Therapy* (Rogers, 1951). There is only one entry under the term "resistance," and that entry directs the reader to "threat." Rogers does not discuss resistance per se, but instead sees what others describe as resistance as the person's response to threat. The core of Rogers's view on resistance is that when an individual perceives experiences that are contradictory to his or her current self-organization, he or she experiences a threat to the organization of the self. The perception of these discrepancies is frightening. In response, defensive behavior or resistance occurs in which experience is denied, distorted, or inadequately symbolized in order to make the experiences seem more congruent with self-organization or to block them from conscious awareness. Resistance, then, occurs as a result of a perceived threat to the consistency and integrity of the self.

Gestalt Therapy

Perls, Hefferline, and Goodman (1951) present an early gestalt therapy perspective on resistance. These authors conceptualized resistance as conflict within the individual that occurred outside of awareness and an avoidance that limited the individual's contact with the self. According to these authors,

[Resistance is a conflict] between one part of your personality and another. Of one part you are aware, the part which sets the tasks and tries to carry them through. Of the other part, the resister, you are less or not at all aware. (pp. 44–45)

Later in their book, these authors write:

In the usual character analysis, the resistances are "attacked," the "defenses" are dissolved, and so forth. But, on the contrary, if the awareness is creative, then these very resistances and defenses—they are really counter-attacks and aggressions against the self—are taken as active expressions of vitality, however neurotic they may be in the total picture. (p. 248)

This view of resistance bears some similarities to Rogers's view, but emphasizes the centrality of conflict among opposing parts of the self. This basic view has been elaborated and extended by Engle and Holiman (2002), Polster and Polster (1973), and Greenberg, Rice, and Elliott (1993).

In a later gestalt view, Polster and Polster (1973) wrote that "what usually passes for resistance is not just a dumb barrier to be removed but a creative force for managing a difficult world" (p. 52). These authors also see resistance as an intrapsychic conflict among aspects of the self. Polster and Polster (1973) also discuss "resistance to contact." They suggest that people manage their energy so that they either make good contact or resist contact with the environment. Healthy functioning depends upon the ability to interact well with the world in order to get what is necessary for continual growth and well-being. Polster and Polster describe manifestations of resistance to contact that consist of ways in which a person can reduce his or her interaction with him- or herself or with the environment. In an example of the former, Greg grew up in a family where emotions (especially "negative" emotions) were not allowed expression. He introjected a belief that emotions are an expression of weakness. As an adult he is not able to express his feelings and is often unable to name what it is that he feels. In an example of the latter, Gretchen periodically has good reasons to be angry with her husband. Rather than confront her husband with her resentments, she, without awareness, "retroflects" her anger. She turns her anger inward and blames herself for all the tension that exists between her and her spouse.

Zinker (1977), Kepner (1987), and others have a somewhat different gestalt model for understanding resistance to contact. They work from a framework that is grounded in what they call the "gestalt cycle" or the "cycle of experience." The cycle is a description of the stages of gestalt formation and completion and proceeds as follows: experiencing a (physical) sensation (e.g., a twitch), giving meaning to it ("I'm anxious"), mobilizing for action, acting, and contacting (the actual experience of the situation. This is followed by withdrawing and an eventual repetition of the cycle.

While Polster and Polster (1973) use the concept of contact boundary disturbances to identify how the "resistance" manifests itself in each individual, Zinker, Kepner, and others use the gestalt cycle to make a similar kind of assessment. A "resistance" can manifest itself at any transition in the gestalt cycle and occurs when the person does not move smoothly through the cycle. For example, a client may have difficulty at the very beginning of the cycle (body sensations are the primary means of grounding ourselves in the environment). She may be unaware of her bodily felt sensations. She does not notice that her jaw is clenched or that she carries a perpetual scowl or that she looks like a coiled spring ready to burst. When she "resists" information provided by the sensations in her body, she denies herself access to an important source of information about her present-moment relationship with her environment. Her needs may go unmet because the sensations are precursors to the development of an understanding of her current needs.

Another person may always be busy, running late, always a little harried, while at the same time complaining that there are some tasks that he wants to achieve but doesn't. That person is in the action stage, but does not move into the essential contact stage that will accomplish the task. Still another may be in the contact stage and resist letting go and moving to the withdrawal stage.

Engle and Holiman (2002) suggest that resistance to awareness serves a self-protective function that keeps the client safe from the anxiety associated with change. According to these authors, resistance manifests itself as a state of ambivalence, reflecting an internal conflict of which the client may be unaware. They further suggest that resistance reflects the client's struggle to balance stability and change, and to avoid the anxiety of change.

Kepner (1987) offers a good summary of the various humanistic-experiential views of resistance. First, he notes that resistance is not a mechanism of the self but is the self itself—expressed in action. This idea derives from the humanistic view of wholeness. All thoughts, feelings, or actions (including resistance) are manifestations of the self. To attempt to "break through" the resistance is an attack on the self. Second, "resistant" expressions of the self operate outside awareness and are "not expressions of choice" (Kepner, 1987, p. 66). They are existential messages from a disowned part of self. Third, and consistent with Perls et al. (1951) and Polster and Polster (1973), Kepner suggests that resistance is an energy or force that is seeking recognition, although in an unsuccessful manner that creates conflict within the person. Fourth, "resistances" do not allow people to interact with the environment in a style that makes it possible for them to get their needs met. Either the person dilutes healthy contact with the environment or makes poor contact with one or more stages of the cycle of gestalt formation and completion.

According to these gestalt views, the goals of treatment are:

- To create a therapy environment in which the "resistance" is respected as an important expression of the self itself. It is not something to be "broken through." Such actions would be tantamount to assaulting the self.
- To reconnect clients with disowned parts of themselves to create a harmonious whole and reduce internal conflict—often through dialogue work.
- To facilitate good contact between the client and the environment.
- To facilitate the client's ability to move appropriately through the natural gestalt formation and completion.
- To work with the anxiety that is inherent in the nature of change.

Motivational interviewing, developed by Miller and Rollnick (1991, 2002) is an integration of the client-centered approach of Carl Rogers with the action orientation of behavior therapy. This approach sees resistance as ambivalence, and will be considered in greater depth in Chapters 8 and 9.

What Changes Are Resisted?

In gestalt and humanistic-experiential approaches, resistance is directed toward awareness of threatening material and toward full contact with the environment. In Rogers's view (1951), resistance primarily consists of the distortions and denials that arise from discrepancies between people's perceived present experience and their overall view of their own self-organization. Gestalt views also emphasize discrepancy and conflict in resistance, but one important aspect of the discrepancy is among aspects of the self—for example, one aspect that tries to change and another that resists change. Often, individuals resist awareness of the aspect that fights against change. Gestalt views also emphasize resistance to contact with the environment in which the individual engages in various ways of avoiding full experience of the environment. This view also emphasizes resistance to moving to the next, natural, and necessary phase of the gestalt cycle.

What Behaviors Define the Presence of Resistance?

In Rogers's view, the behaviors that define resistance consist primarily of denials or distortions of experience that are incompatible with the perceived self. For example, a man who perceives himself as kind and gentle may deny or distort feelings of intense anger because they are inconsistent with his self-view.

Gestalt views primarily emphasize behaviors that indicate ambivalence, reflecting an internal conflict among aspects of the self. This may be seen in statements like "Yes, but . . . " or in discrepancies between a person's verbal and nonverbal behaviors. Other behaviors signaling the presence of resistance involve the various styles described by Polster and Polster (1973) in which individuals resist direct contact with their environment. For Kepner (1987), resistance is being stuck in a particular stage of the gestalt cycle.

Why Is Resistance Occurring?

As with other approaches, resistance in humanistic-experiential therapies is a response to anxiety or threat. It is the nature of the hypothesized threat that distinguishes this approach from the others. Resistance occurs mainly because of perceptions that are inconsistent with the individual's view of his or her self-organization. This is true for both client-centered therapy and gestalt therapy. However, gestalt therapy emphasizes that the part of the person that resists change is the threatening one that must be kept out of awareness, but nonetheless influences the person and creates an internal conflict of which the person is unaware.

How Do Humanistic-Experiential Approaches Work with Resistance in Clinical Practice?

According to Rogers (1951), change occurs because the therapist accepts and values aspects of the client that the client finds threatening and keeps from his or her own awareness. This makes it possible for the client to become aware of and accept them as well. The client is able to internalize the therapist's attitudes and calmly approach the formerly threatening awareness of self. Rogers writes: "If the relationship is not adequate to provide this sense of safety, or if the denied experiences are too threatening, then the client may revise his concept of self in a defensive fashion" (1951, p. 194).

Gestalt approaches also emphasize the therapist's acceptance of threatening aspects of the client's experience, but use "experiments" to help clients integrate those aspects into their self-concept. According to Engle and Holiman (2002), the purpose of these experiments is to increase awareness, to make contact with discrepancies, and to resolve them. Common forms of experiments are two-chair and empty-chair experiments, both of which have been described by Greenberg et al. (1993). These are discussed more fully in subsequent chapters.

FAMILY SYSTEMS PERSPECTIVES ON RESISTANCE

Nichols and Schwartz (2001) suggested that early family therapists interpreted resistance as *homeostasis*, or a force that opposed change in systems. They commented that more recent family theories recognize that all human systems are reluctant to make changes that involve risk. These theories recognize that families should resist change until they are sure that the therapist can be trusted and that change is safe. The view shifted from resistance as a kind of stubbornness implied by homeostasis to a view of resistance as having a self-protective function.

A number of family therapy approaches are basically extensions of constructs and strategies from the respective individual therapy to families. These include psychoanalytic, cognitive-behavioral, and experiential family therapies. The views of resistance in these family approaches closely parallel those of the respective individual therapies. This brief review focuses on three unique family approaches: structural, systemic, and the integrative approach of Anderson and Stewart (1983). There are considerable differences in the ways that these therapies approach resistance. Whether therapists attempt to avoid, overcome, or use resistance to produce change depends on their theoretical orientation.

Structural Approaches

The structural approach to family therapy (Aponte & Van Deusen, 1981; Minuchin, 1974; Minuchin & Fishman, 1981) is primarily concerned with family structure, which includes boundaries, subsystems, and the relationships among them, as well as the relationship of the family to the broader environment in which it functions. The symptoms of an individual family member are viewed as a failure of the family to adjust to the changing demands of its members and are maintained by the ways in which family members relate to one another. Structural approaches emphasize homeostatic mechanisms by which the family tends to retain its current way of functioning as a system, seeking to maintain the status quo, even though it may be maladaptive.

This homeostasis is based on the family's implicit rules that govern how family members interrelate. It is these rules that tend to be self-perpetuating and which the family as a system seeks to maintain. It is also these rules that need to be changed to effectively change psychopathology in the family and its members.

The structural approach suggests that an individual's symptoms should be examined in the context of family interactional patterns. A change in the family organization or structure must take place before an individual's symptoms can change.

Structural approaches use a variety of techniques that are aimed at changing the structure of the family. These include (but are not limited to) reframing, or attributing a different meaning to a behavior so that it will be seen differently by the family; unbalancing—for example, by siding with one member of the family in order to change relationships within the system; and shaping competence or highlighting positive behaviors.

Strategic Approaches

Strategic family therapists (Bateson, Jackson, Haley, & Weakland, 1956; Haley, 1976) view resistance as a central concept in working with families. They place more emphasis on symptoms than do structural family therapists and see symptoms as an expression of the fact that the person is stuck in a situation and cannot get out of it.

Like those who follow the structural approach, these therapists assume that families operate with repetitive modes of interactions among family members that define the implicit rules of functioning of the family. In dysfunctional families, these rules have not changed to meet changing circumstances or the changed needs of individual family members. Instead, dysfunctional families respond to these demands by the repetition or escalation of family mechanisms that are not successful in solving the problems.

Strategic therapists believe that changes in the ways that members of the family act must precede changes in perceptions and feelings. There are numerous techniques that strategic therapists employ to effect change. Some of the major ones are described below:

1. Reframing, in which a different interpretation is given to a family's situation or behavior. It results in a changed meaning that may reduce resistance. For example, the aloofness of a family member may be reframed as his attempt to cautiously protect the family from outsiders. It may be easier to reach and work with this individual when his behavior is reframed this way rather than as defensiveness.

2. Therapist directives to the family to behave differently. Straightforward directives are useful for the family members who tend to do what the therapist asks, but paradoxical directives are more effective for those who tend to resist therapist directives.

3. Paradoxical interventions—attempts to induce change by discouraging it (Rohrbaugh, Tennen, Press, & White, 1981; Tennen, Rohrbaugh, Press, & White, 1981; Shoham, Trost, & Rohrbaugh, 2004). One of the most common involves various forms of "prescribing the symptom." Such interventions may arouse reactance, leading the client or family to do the opposite of the directive, thereby changing. Such interventions are used to help a person or family abandon dysfunctional behavior. The purpose is to unbalance a system that has become stuck.

Anderson and Stewart's Pragmatic Approach

Anderson and Stewart (1983) present what they call a "pragmatic" view of resistance in family therapy, acknowledging the diversity in the views that exist. They draw from several different theories in their integrative approach. Anderson and Stewart suggest that resistance arises from an interaction of three parts of the therapeutic system: the therapist, the family, and the health service delivery system. While they suggest that these three parts interact, they consider each part and its potential contributions to resistance separately.

From the perspective of the family, Anderson and Stewart suggest that the heritage that each spouse brings to a relationship contributes to ways of responding in the family that become habitual. Such patterns are predictable and safe. Resistance to change can arise from unexamined beliefs about family heritages and the relative rigidity of such beliefs.

Anderson and Stewart also suggest that the major sources of family resistance stem from *anxiety about change* and *striving for stability*. Change is associated with anxiety because it may threaten familiar and secure, albeit dysfunctional, patterns of interaction. In addition, family members will resist changing patterns of behavior that are central to their sense of personal identity, and may respond to attempts to change them with resistance when those change attempts are perceived as threats to the family's freedom.

What Changes Are Resisted?

The conceptualization of most of the family systems approaches reviewed here ist that families resist attempts to change implicit family rules that dictate how members respond to one another. In this sense, *it is a change in the structure and rules of the family that is resisted*, even though these may have outlived their usefulness and may be contributing to pathological functioning in the family and/or its individual members. In addition, *changes in the symptoms of one of the members may also be resisted* because of the role that the family member and his or her symptoms play in the family.

What Behaviors Define the Presence of Resistance?

Gladding (1995) describes a number of manifestations of resistance in family therapy including members' attempts to control sessions, missing sessions, silence during sessions, refusals of members to talk to each other in sessions, expressions of hostility, rationalizing, insisting that one family member is the problem, challenging the therapist's competence, and failure to do homework. In addition, repetitive, rigid, stereotyped, and dysfunctional patterns of interaction in the family constitute major indicators of resistance.

Why Is Resistance Occurring?

Two central and complementary reasons for resistance in family systems theories are *maintenance of the status quo and fear of change*. These occur because change may threaten the identities and security of individual family members and family members may respond with reactance, opposing change in an attempt to assert their freedom and autonomy from influence.

How Do Family Therapists Work with Resistance in Clinical Practice?

For the most part, structural family therapists see *resistance as an obstacle to be avoided or overcome* by the therapist so that change can occur. The therapist's role is to enter into the family system and challenge it in various ways in order to effect change. Minuchin's approach (cited in Nichols & Schwartz, 2001) is to join families and win them over and accommodate them. Doing this gives the family therapist the leverage to use confrontational techniques to restructure the family. Therapy occurs by alternately challenging the family and then rejoining it. Hoffman (1981), a well-known strategic family therapist, suggests that "resistance can be a positive force that generates the momentum for change, as in paradoxical interventions" (p. 348). Strategic therapists also use relabeling or reframing to change their meanings in the family context so that they are perceived as less negative.

Anderson and Stewart (1983) devote an entire book to strategies for working with resistance in family therapy, drawing from other approaches as well as from their own innovations. While a thorough review of their thoughtful work is beyond the scope of this chapter, their approach is noteworthy in two ways. First, while they focus on resistance from the family, they also look at resistance as possibly arising from the health care delivery system and the therapist, as well as the interactions of these with each other and with the family. These authors also present an analysis of resistance and where and how it may appear in family therapy over the entire course of the therapy, starting with the first phone call and through ongoing treatment.

REACTANCE THEORY

Reactance theory is not a theory of resistance per se, nor does it have a particular therapeutic approach associated with it. It is a social psychological theory developed originally by Jack Brehm (1966; Brehm & Brehm, 1981) and initially extended to clinical psychology by Sharon Brehm (1976). There is a large body of research associated with reactance theory (see Brehm & Brehm, 1981; Wright, Greenberg, & Brehm, 2004). A number of publications on resistance have drawn on reactance theory (e.g., Beutler et al., 2002; Dowd & Wallbrown, 1993; Shoham-Salomon, Avner, & Neeman, 1989; Shoham et al., 2004). It is considered in this chapter because we believe that it has a great deal of potential for understanding certain aspects of resistance and how to work with it.

Before considering reactance, we need to examine what J. Brehm (1966) calls "free behaviors." These are behaviors that a person can choose to engage in or not, now or in the future. A central tenet of reactance theory is that "a person will experience psychological reactance whenever any of his or her free behaviors are eliminated or threatened with elimination" (S. Brehm, 1976). Reactance may be induced by others (e.g., when they give us orders) or it may be self-imposed. J. Brehm (1966) gives the example of decision making to illustrate a self-imposed threat to freedom. When we make a decision and choose one alternative over the other, we often limit our ability to have the less preferred one. We suggest that there is another type of self-imposed reactance that is highly relevant to psychotherapy. This occurs when we limit our own freedom. For example, a dieter must limit the amount that he or she eats. Dieters take from themselves the freedom to eat whatever they want in quantities they want. More generally, the "shoulds" that we each carry with us can be seen as self-imposed threats to our freedom and may elicit reactance as well.

Reactance arousal is a motivational state that directs us toward the restoration of the threatened or eliminated freedom. While there are several ways in which reactance may be manifested (S. Brehm, 1976, p. 19), the most common are noncompliance and oppositional behavior. When given an order (by others or by our own self-directives, or "shoulds"), our reactance is aroused. We may choose not to comply or even do the opposite in order to reduce reactance. There is a considerable body of research relevant to therapy that supports the idea that people are less likely to comply when given strong directives than they are when a request is made in a nonauthoritarian way (Patterson & Chamberlain, 1994; Miller, Benefield, & Tonigan, 1993).

The Brehms clearly conceptualized reactance as a state. Dowd and his associates (e.g., Dowd, Milne, & Wise, 1991; Dowd, Wallbrown, Sanders, & Yesenosky, 1994) also saw the potential of reactance for understanding resistance in psychotherapy. Dowd developed a self-report measure called the Therapeutic Reactance Scale. However, he conceptualized reactance as a cross-situational trait rather than as a situation-specific state. Psychotherapy research that has treated reactance as a client trait has typically measured it as a pretreatment individual difference variable so that its effects on outcome could be evaluated. Shoham et al. (2004) have challenged the notion of reactance as a trait. They have argued convincingly that research support for reactance as a trait has been mixed at best. Instead, they cogently argue that research needs to return to studying reactance as a state. They have conducted studies that provide strong support for this view (e.g., Shoham, Bootzin, Rohrbaugh, & Urry, 1996; Shoham-Salomon et al., 1989) and reviewed others.

Reactance has been employed as one explanation of the effects of "paradoxical interventions" in therapy (Rohrbaugh et al., 1981; Tennen et al., 1981). *Paradoxical interventions* attempt to induce change by discouraging it (Shoham et al., 2004). The most common approach is to prescribe the symptom—for example, suggesting to a depressed person that he or she should take care of him- or herself by staying at home and resting. Since such a directive potentially limits the client's free behaviors, he or she may be more likely to be active outside of the home in order to defy the directive and reduce reactance. In the process, he or she also engages in behaviors that may help reduce depression.

What Changes Are Resisted?

We resist attempts by others and by ourselves to limit our freedom.

What Behaviors Define the Presence of Resistance?

Most often, the behaviors reflect noncompliance with directives or oppositional behaviors.

Why Is Resistance Occurring?

1. To reduce the motivational state of reactance.
2. To restore the freedoms that we perceive to be eliminated, limited, or threatened.

How Does Reactance Theory Work with Resistance in Clinical Practice?

While there is no specific therapeutic approach associated with react-ance theory, it follows from the theory that directiveness on the part of the therapist will elicit reactance/resistance, while supportive/empathic interventions are more likely to elicit change.

CONSTRUCTIVIST THEORY

Constructivist theory is broadly integrative, incorporating aspects of the major schools of psychotherapy as well as insights from other scientific fields. It is really a family of theories (Mahoney & Marquis, 2002) that share certain assumptions in common:

- The importance of human agency, or the active role we play in our own lives; the importance of ordering processes that are "pri-marily emotional, tacit, and categorical (they depend on con-trasts), and they are the essence of meaning making" (Mahoney, 2003, p. 5).
- The centrality of the phenomenological sense of selfhood or per-sonal identity.
- The influence of social–symbolic processes.
- Principles of dynamic dialectical development involving cycles and spirals of experiencing.

The constructivist view is strongly based in a phenomenological perspective in which the reality as perceived by the individual is the one that needs to be respected and understood. Mahoney and Neimeyer have been two of the leading figures in applying it to psychotherapy (Mahoney, 1991, 2003; Neimeyer & Mahoney, 1995).

In his 1991 book, Mahoney examined reasons for resistance that seemed to cut across various theories and therapies. These included:

- Motivated avoidance
- Motivational deficit
- Ambivalent choice
- Reactance
- Self-protection

While the constructivist view incorporates all of these, it places greatest emphasis on the protection of the self in the face of challenges to change. Mahoney (1993) suggested that continuity (i.e., lack of change) and structure are basic themes of our existence. He suggested that there is some adaptive, value to our resisting change in core ordering processes. In part, old patterns resist change because they are familiar and maintain the consistency and integrity of the self, even if their consequences are painful. Mahoney (2003) suggests that "old habits often become sanctuaries" (p. 173). Mahoney further suggests that many of the problematic patterns and symptoms that people try to change are attempted short-term solutions to problems of pain and meaning.

For these reasons, constructivist therapy does not try to eliminate or break through resistance. Instead, it works *with* rather than *against* resistance, and sees it as having meaning and serving functions for the individual. Not pushing for change, but instead conveying compassion and empathy for the role that resistance plays for the person, is a basic component of the constructivist approach to working with resistance. Mahoney suggests that pushing to change in the face of resistance often fails and reinforces the resistance. The less we push ourselves or others to change, the more likely we are to change—this point of view is similar to humanistic and motivational interviewing positions. This is because change is frightening and the status quo provides security and consistency, as well as a partial solution to problems in our lives. Constructivist therapy deals with resistance by respecting the importance and functions of staying the same while at the same time inviting the person to consider change.

What Changes Are Resisted?

In the constructivist view, the most basic changes that are resisted are those that relate to the self-system.

What Behaviors Define the Presence of Resistance?

These are not specified but would likely be similar to those of other theories, especially humanistic-experiential ones.

Why Is Resistance Occurring?

While resistance may occur for a variety of reasons as listed above, constructivist views stress that resistance is to be expected as part of the oscillating change process. *Resistance to change in the self-system occurs because the status quo provides security and consistency and change threatens the integrity of the self.*

How Does Constructivist Therapy Work with Resistance in Clinical Practice?

Constructivist therapists convey empathy and compassion for the person's desires not to change, respecting the reasons the person has for resisting change. They also invite the person to change at his or her own pace, rather than trying to force change.

SYNTHESIS

Our review of theories of resistance has revealed significant commonalities as well as differences across the theories discussed.[2] Any attempt to abstract some of the main commonalities across such diverse points of view is fraught with difficulties of subjectivity and selectivity. We will nonetheless attempt to abstract what we consider to be some of the main themes in each area in order to set the stage for our own integrative approach, which we present in Chapter 3.

Below, we list what we consider to be some of the main themes that emerged from our review. Consistent with a common-factors point of view (Arkowitz, 1997), we think such an abstraction has the potential benefit of identifying some useful information about resistance that may get lost in the jargon and specifics of each approach. Here is our synthesis:

What Changes Are Resisted?
- Changes in pathogenic beliefs and schemas.
- Changes in repetitive and maladaptive interpersonal patterns.
- Awareness of painful thoughts or feelings that are discrepant with current views of the self.

---

[2]The Appendix presents a comparison across the six theories in terms of how they address the four questions.

- Implicit or explicit suggestions to comply with the procedures of the therapy during the session and in homework between sessions.
- Change in the status quo.

What Behaviors Define the Presence of Resistance?

- Avoidance of painful insights or awareness of feelings.
- Denials or distortions of experience that are incompatible with the perceived self.
- Continued engagement in long-term repetitive and maladaptive interpersonal patterns.
- Noncompliance with either in-session or between-session procedures, assignments, or experiments.
- Behaviors that indicate ambivalence, reflecting an internal conflict among aspects of the self.

Why Is Resistance Occurring?

- Anxiety reduction through avoidance of anxiety-generating insight into or awareness of one's painful thoughts or feelings.
- "Diablos conocidos" (familiar devils)—the security and predictability of the familiar. Change in the self-system is resisted because the status quo provides security and consistency and change threatens the integrity of the self.
- Fear of change.
- Pathogenic beliefs that maintain symptomatic behaviors.
- Vicious cycles in which the person's beliefs carried forward from earlier in life are confirmed by the way the person perceives and structures his or her world in the present.
- Secondary gain in which the person receives benefit from the symptomatic behavior.
- Therapist deficiencies (e.g., inadequate case conceptualization).
- Client characteristics (e.g., poor impulse control).
- Problems in the relationship between therapist and client.
- Others in the person's life (e.g., family members) may have an investment in the client not changing.
- Ambivalence or internal conflict in which a part of the self that wishes to change is in conflict with a part that resists change.

- To reduce the motivational state of reactance and to restore the freedoms that we perceive to be eliminated, limited, or threatened by a directive.

How Do the Approaches Reviewed Work with Resistance in Clinical Practice?

- Therapist comments and interpretations that identify defensive avoidance and repetitive interpersonal patterns in and out of therapy and link them to early conflictual experiences.
- Corrective emotional experience in which the therapist does not respond as the client expected, leading the client to question the need to engage in these patterns of behavior.
- Discovering and changing conditions that may maintain non-compliant behaviors (e.g., eliciting stimuli and reinforcers).
- Teaching the client to correct inaccurate and distorted thoughts and beliefs and to modify schemas underlying the resistance through directive interventions (persuasion or directives) or through collaboratively examining distorted thoughts using thought records and/or between-session experiments to test the accuracy of the thoughts.
- Therapist attitudes toward the client that convey safety and acceptance and allow the client to more easily become aware of and work with threatening awareness of self.
- Experiments (e.g., two-chair technique) to help clients become more aware of and to integrate aspects of the self that have been out of awareness and that contribute to resistance.
- Therapist entering into the family system and challenging it in various ways that include directives, reframing, and paradoxical interventions.
- Using a supportive and relatively nondirective style to show empathy for the difficulties of changing and to avoid arousing reactance.

SUMMARY

In this chapter, we compared four major theories of resistance—psychoanalytic, cognitive-behavioral, humanistic-experiential, and family systems—and two more recent points of view on resistance—

reactance theory and constructivist approaches. The theories were compared on their understanding of what is resisted, what behaviors define the presence of resistance, why is resistance occurring, and how do the different therapies work with resistance. While there clearly are differences among some of them, there are also a number of common themes that cut across several of these points of view. The chapter concluded with a synthesis of these common themes as they relate to each of the four questions.

CHAPTER 3

An Integrative Model
of Resistant Ambivalence

In this chapter, we present an integrative model for understanding and working with resistance. We suggest that many, perhaps even most, instances of resistance can be understood as ambivalence in which some behavioral indicators point *toward* change while others point *away* from change. The client who seeks out therapy and verbally expresses a wish to change is obviously manifesting indicators regarding a desire to change. However, if that same client cancels many sessions and engages the therapist in ways that appear to frustrate attempts to help him or her change, then we may infer ambivalence. We will be dealing with instances in which people:

- Express some desire to change.
- Indicate that they believe that change will improve their lives.
- Believe that effective strategies for change are available to them.
- Have adequate information about executing those strategies, but nonetheless don't employ them sufficiently for change to occur.
- Experience accompanying negative affect.

The assumptions of our model draw heavily from the common themes that emerged from our review of theories of resistance in Chapter 2. A general description of the model that we are proposing is that *resistant ambivalence derives from discrepancies among self-schemas relevant to change.* The model is integrative, that is, it draws from existing theories of resistance as well as from recent research and theory on social cognition and self-schemas.

The assumptions of our model are:

- Many instances of resistance can be understood as ambivalence.
- Resistant ambivalence is most commonly manifested as defensive avoidance, noncompliance, and the repetitive pattern of interpersonal behaviors that cause lack of gratification or distress.
- The data on resistant ambivalence provide important information that can best be understood from the client's perspective.
- Resistant ambivalence is intrapersonal and reflects discrepancies among self-schemas relevant to change—that is, those that are associated with movement toward change and those that are associated with movement away from change.
- People may not be fully aware of their self-schemas or the discrepancies among them that cause resistant ambivalence.
- Resistant ambivalence is interpersonal and needs to be understood in the interpersonal context in which it occurs.
- Change is often resisted because it is associated with a sense of unpredictability and uncontrollability, while the status quo is embraced because it is perceived as relatively safe.
- Resistant ambivalence can best be understood as a state rather than as a trait.
- Approaches to resistant ambivalence that provide empathy and support are more likely to facilitate change than more directive approaches.

In the remainder of this chapter, we discuss and elaborate on each of these assumptions.

1. *Many instances of resistance can be understood as ambivalence.* Ambivalence occurs when there is some desire to change but other indicators point away from change. We believe that resistant ambivalence involves a continual process of approaching and avoiding change. However, there are two other instances in which people may be labeled "resistant" but where there seems to be no ambivalence present. In the first, the person shows no desire to change, but friends and family express strong desires for him or her to change. Many alcoholics, drug addicts, and people with eating disorders often show no desire to change (although their attitudes can change over time). Also, those diagnosed with

certain disorders (e.g., antisocial and paranoid personality disorders) and clients with bipolar disorder in a hypomanic or manic state often show no desire to change. A second instance of resistance that does not involve any apparent ambivalence is when a person wants to change but doesn't know how to change. People who are unaware of the availability of effective treatments for their problem fall into this category.

2. *Resistant ambivalence manifests itself as defensive avoidance, noncompliance, or a repetitive pattern of maladaptive interpersonal behaviors.* When these patterns of behavior are seen in therapy, they are usually of the "yes, but . . . " variety. The "yes" is reflected in clients' expressed desires to approach anxiety-laden thoughts and feelings, to do the homework, and to change those interpersonal behavior patterns. The "but" expresses the other side of the ambivalence that moves the person away from those changes.

3. *The data concerning resistant ambivalence provide important information that can be best understood from the client's perspective.* These reasons often relate to the person's hopes, fears, and desires about change. The data addressing resistance are informative about important aspects of the person's current functioning and, in Schwartz's (1991) terms, may be considered to be "friendly data." That is, our resistances can be seen as informative about ourselves, even if they make us aware of information that is unpleasant. Schwartz (1991) pointed out that data is "friendly" since information per se is always potentially valuable and never in itself harmful.

This point can be illustrated by the case of a middle-aged man who was referred to us by his family physician. The man had diabetes and very high blood pressure. His blood pressure remained high despite his regular use of medication for the condition. He was less compliant regarding the medication for his diabetes. Moreover, he did not follow any of his doctor's recommendations for controlling his diet and starting on an exercise program. His weight was in the normal range, but he persisted in eating foods that contributed to his high blood pressure and high glucose levels. He was stably married and had three children. He described his family life and job as both "Okay." His family was upset with his noncompliant behaviors: they were afraid that he would suffer an early death. Why would anyone with an apparently satisfying life act in ways that appear self-destructive? From the external perspective of his family, he was behaving foolishly and irrationally. Yet our assessment emphasized his perspective rather than theirs. From his point of view, there were many good reasons for acting as he did. He stated that while most important things in his life were "okay," none were especially interesting or exciting. The area of his life that was most pleasurable for him was eating foods he enjoyed, like ribs. Most of what he enjoyed eating was also bad for his health. In addition, he stated that he didn't want to live his later years as his parents had done. He described their senior years as obsessed with diet, medication, and health. He stated that he would rather "go out of this life having a good time" than live like his parents did. These are the thoughts that determined his noncompliant behavior, thoughts that needed to be understood and respected if change was going to occur.

Information about resistance can also potentially be used to facilitate change. We may not like the fact of our resistances, but our resistant patterns inform us of aspects of ourselves relating to change to which we need to attend. Contrast this position with others that argue that resistance is an annoying obstacle to be overcome by paradox, contingencies, or other means.

In the integrative framework presented here, resistant ambivalence is not simply an obstacle to overcome by the therapist and the client, but a reflection of the individual's hopes, desires, wishes, and fears. In order to help people change, we need to understand and respect these basic aspects of who they are and how they see the pros and cons of change. We need to understand how they feel and think from within their own perspectives rather than from an external point of view. For example, a spouse or family member usually can only see how change will be positive and cannot readily see or appreciate the individual's reasons for not changing. An alcoholic may resist change because giving up drinking involves giving up one of the only pleasures and releases in his stressful life, as well as giving up his drinking friends. But family and friends are so focused on the negative impact of drinking on the person's health, work, and relationships that they often don't appreciate the significance of the sacrifices that change would involve. Such sacrifice can only be appreciated from the person's frame of reference and not from the external perspective of another.

The important data about resistance involve the person's perceptions and mental representations that relate to change. We are primarily concerned with perceptions and only secondarily concerned with the "reality" of the cues and situations to which he or she is responding. For example, if a man perceives that attempting to change will be difficult, painful, or unsuccessful, he probably won't attempt to change, even if his perceptions are incorrect. Measuring and understanding the intrapersonal mental representations relating to change is central to the present model since our mental representations influence whether or not we will attempt change. Moreover, they may do so in a variety of ways.

4. *Resistant ambivalence is intrapersonal and reflects discrepancies among self-schemas relevant to change.* Theory and research in personality and the cognitive sciences (e.g., Higgins, 1996; Markus & Nurius, 1986) have emphasized the concept of self-schemas. Fiske and Taylor (1991) define *self-schemas* as "cognitive-affective structures that represent one's experience in a given domain. They organize and direct the processing of information relevant to the self-schema" (1991, pp. 182–183). Self-schemas are generalizations about the self in particular behavioral domains (Markus & Nurius, 1986; Stein & Markus, 1994) that develop from categorizations and evaluations of the self made by oneself and others. These domains may relate to our hopes, fears, and potentials. The term "self-schemas" refers to different aspects of what Markus and Nurius (1986) have called our "possible selves," and differs from an overall one-dimensional self-concept.

Self-schemas have an emotional component as well as an action tendency. For example, if part of our "Desired Self" schema is to be more physically active, then our mood will become more positive as we become more active or more negative if we neglect physical exercise.

Understanding those self-schemas that may relate to change can help us to understand the phenomena of resistance. More specifically, we are suggesting that interactions and discrepancies among different self-schemas relating to change will determine ambivalence, or what we call resistance. Thus, an awareness of what we desire for ourselves may be useful, but may constitute only a partial understanding of resistance. We may better understand resistance when we look at how our desires relate to our fears, "shoulds," or even our estimates of what we can attain for ourselves. Higgins (1996) and Oyserman and Markus (1990) have also emphasized the importance of understanding the relationships among our different self-schemas to understand and predict emotion and behavior.

5. *People may not be fully aware of their self-schemas or of the discrepancies among them that cause resistant ambivalence.* Recent research in the cognitive sciences (e.g., Schacter, 1995) has found evidence for what Kihlstrom (1987) has called the "cognitive unconscious," or cognitive processes and contents that may be out of awareness but that nonetheless

may influence us nonetheless (Fiske & Taylor, 1991). People may be unaware of the specific personal characteristics that are included in their different self-schemas until they are asked to list them, and they may be even less aware of interactions or discrepancies among their self-schemas. The assumption that important processes about resistance take place outside of conscious awareness is a fundamental one, not only in psychoanalytic views, but in gestalt-experiential and cognitive-behavioral approaches too

6. *Since resistant ambivalence is interpersonal, it needs to be understood in the interpersonal context in which it occurs.* While an intrapersonal perspective is important in understanding ambivalence, it is just as important to understand the interpersonal context in which it occurs. Often resistance is a reaction to perceived attempts by others to limit our freedoms, as described by reactance theory. In addition, the consistent finding in the psychotherapy literature that a positive therapeutic relationship is one of the most important predictors of therapeutic change (e.g., Lambert & Barley, 2002) suggests once again that the quality of the therapist–client relationship is a potentially important determinant of resistant ambivalence.

7. *Change is often resisted because it is associated with a sense of unpredictability and uncontrollability while the status quo is associated with a sense of relative safety.* It's interesting to note that this point comes up in almost every theory of resistance, although it is often couched in different theoretical languages. Barlow (2002) has reviewed literature that points to the significance of perceptions of unpredictability and uncontrollability in anxiety and anxiety disorders. According to Barlow, the more that we perceive our world as unpredictable and uncontrollable, the more anxiety we experience. Although we approach change because we believe that it will have obvious benefits such as reduced distress and better relationships, it makes our world less stable and secure. For example, a depressed person who makes efforts to change his or her depression may also realize that if he or she is successful in doing so he or she will then have to face the interpersonal or occupational stresses that may have contributed to his or her depression in the first place. Similarly, a person with panic disorder and agoraphobia who participates in exposure therapy cannot be sure that exposing him- or herself to new situations will prevent all subsequent panic attacks. Further, if the agoraphobia is eliminated, his or her relationships with others need to change so that the client is no longer so dependent on others. In such cases, change is associ-

ated with giving up the feelings of safety and security that the agoraphobic experienced through the presence of others who accompanied him or her when he or she went out.

8. *Resistant ambivalence can best be understood as a state rather than as a trait.* It seems obvious that people can be ambivalent about some areas of their lives but not about other areas. For this reason, we believe that ambivalence is best viewed as a situation-specific state rather than as a cross-situational trait. Research reviewed by Shoham, Trost, and Rohrbaugh (2004) supports a similar view of reactance as state versus trait. While treating reactance as a trait has yielded some positive results, overall results of such studies have been quite mixed. By contrast, when reactance is treated as a state, findings have been clearer and more consistent (Shoham et al., 2004). We recognize that there may be individual differences in how many situations elicit ambivalence, and also that there may be some individuals who are highly ambivalent across situations. But we prefer to let data show that this is the case rather than making an a priori assumption that there are traits of ambivalence and reactance.

9. *Approaches based on empathy and support are more likely to facilitate change than more directive approaches.* Numerous studies support the conclusion that more directive attempts to get someone to change are less likely to work than those that are based on empathy and support (Burns & Nolen-Hoeksma, 1991, 1992; Miller, Benefield, & Tonigan, 1993; Patterson & Chamberlain, 1994). It is often true that the more we try to change people, the less they actually change. It is also true that the less we try to change them and the more we try to provide empathy and support in their own attempts to change, the more likely they are to change. This is a crucial point. Miller and Rollnick (1991, 2002) have based their motivational interviewing on it. They suggest that the more we advocate for change in another person, the less likely that person is to change. As a result, Miller and Rollnick (2002) focus their approach on ways to increase the other person's intrinsic motivation to change rather than on direct therapeutic attempts to effect change.

This point is a key assumption of most humanistic-experiential approaches, but is much less a part of CBT, psychoanalytic, and (some) family systems approaches. In the latter three approaches, the therapist usually has a clearly identified role as change advocate. Given the interpersonal determinants of resistant ambivalence discussed above, the fact that these therapists so clearly identify with that role may be one significant reason for the occurrence of resistance or noncompliance in those therapies.

SELF-SCHEMAS RELATING TO RESISTANCE AND NONCOMPLIANCE

Which self-schemas are most relevant to understanding resistance? Our model doesn't specify any particular ones, but instead directs the therapist to look for discrepancies or conflicts among whatever schemas lie beneath resistant ambivalent behavior. However, our own clinical experience and the literature suggest certain schemas and discrepancies that we have observed in many cases. We present these as illustrative rather than as exhaustive.

Drawing from conceptualizations of resistance in the theories discussed in the previous chapter, as well as from research in social cognition (Higgins, 1996; Markus & Nurius, 1986; Van Hook & Higgins, 1988) and in reactance theory (Brehm & Brehm, 1981), we have focused our work thus far on five schemas: the Actual Self, the Desired Self, the Should Self, the Feared Self, and the Reactant Self.

AMBIVALENCE AND RESISTANCE AS DISCREPANCIES AMONG SELF SCHEMAS

In the empirical literature on social cognition, several prominent researchers have demonstrated that it is the relationships among self-schemas that cause emotions and ambivalence, rather than the simple presence or absence of a single self-schema. For example, Higgins and his colleagues have developed a measure called the Selves Questionnaire that we discuss in Chapter 4, and they have done a number of studies consistent with the idea that discrepancies between Actual and Should Selves are associated with anxiety and discrepancies between Actual and Desired Selves are associated with dejection/depression (Higgins, 1987; Higgins, Bond, Klein, & Strauman, 1986; Higgins, Klein, & Strauman, 1985; Strauman, 1992).

Consistent with the work of Higgins and his colleagues, we assume that it is not the existence of a single schema that provides the most useful information about ambivalence and resistance, but the interactions among them. It is when the action tendencies associated with different schemas (see Greenberg et al., 1993) pull us in different directions that we act in ambivalent and resistant ways. Some of the discrepancies that we have observed when people act in resistant and ambivalent ways are the following.

Discrepancies between Desired and Should Selves

When the characteristics of the person we want or desire to be are discrepant with the characteristics of the kind of person that we believe we are, ambivalent resistance will result. Since self-schemas are hypothesized to have incentive values, and since the different self-schemas move clients in different directions, therapists may expect to see ambivalent or resistant behavior in their clients when such discrepancies occur. For example, one client expressed a desire to be more relaxed and carefree, but also believed that he should be more ambitious, hard-driving, and successful. In this case, the more he takes time to relax, the more uncomfortable he will feel for not doing what he "should" be doing. However, the more he works, the more uncomfortable he will feel because he is not doing what he "wants" to do. This results in a pattern of approach and avoidance to both work and relaxation. Consistent with this view, Van Hook and Higgins (1988) found that subjects who had discrepancies between their Should and their Desired Selves (or what Higgins and his associates call the "Ought" and the "Ideal" Selves, respectively) were more likely to experience confusion-related emotions (e.g., to be unsure of self or self's goals, muddled, or confused about identity). This confusion is related to what Van Hook and Higgins (1988) refer to as a "double approach–avoidance conflict" (see Heilizer, 1977) in which each end state has both a positive and a negative valence. The more one meets one goal, the more one fails to meet the other, resulting in positive feelings from the former and negative feelings from the latter.

Discrepancies between Desired and Feared Selves

In some instances, resistance to change may result from our being afraid of achieving what we desire to achieve. In other words, the person both desires and fears change, which leads to a pattern of ambivalence and resistance. I (DEE) worked with a young man who sought therapy in order to lose weight so that he could more easily meet women and have an intimate relationship (his Desired Self). As we began to focus on weight loss, he began to exhibit a pattern of ambivalence. He neglected our agreed-upon between-sessions exercises of self-monitoring his food intake and weighing himself weekly. When I discussed this with him, his fears relating to successfully losing weight and then having to deal with sexuality, sexual performance, and intimacy emerged. Essentially, the thought of attaining his Desired Self (being thinner, having a relationship with a woman) activated his Feared Self (being sexually inadequate, unable to deal with an intimate relationship), resulting in ambivalent resistance.

Discrepancies between Should and Reactant Selves

In this discrepancy, the movement toward achieving the characteristics of the Should Self is countered by a Reactant Self that responds negatively and oppositionally to those directives. While Brehm and Brehm (1981) and others who have written about reactance have emphasized its *interpersonal* determinants, we believe that reactance is a phenomenon that can also occur *intrapersonally,* that is, when we are the one who both gives and receives the directive.

Just as directives from others may be perceived as limiting our freedoms, directives from ourselves (our "shoulds") are also experienced as limiting our freedom and may elicit reactance and oppositional behavior. A few years ago, I (HA) decided to begin a vegetarian diet. Even though I typically ate meat only once every few weeks, I chose to totally eliminate meat from my diet by telling myself, in effect, "You should not eat meat any more." In the next few weeks, my craving for meat drastically increased and I ate more meat while on this diet than before I started it. I finally decided that I would eat less meat by allowing myself to eat meat sometimes than by restricting my freedom to do so. Another example of such internal reactance comes from the work of social psychologist Daniel Wegner (1989). To illustrate, the reader might try the following exercise: "Right after you read this, close your eyes and tell yourself *not* to think of a pink elephant." Very likely, you found yourself thinking of a pink elephant. Wegner has labeled this and similar phenomena as "ironic processes of mental control." These processes may be seen in clients with panic disorder whose directive to themselves to relax often leads to an escalation of their panic. Similarly, in obsessive–compulsive disorder, it appears that the more the person tries not to think about his or her obsessive thoughts, the more he or she does so.

There are many other self-schema discrepancies that we have seen in our clinical work with ambivalence, but these three have been by far the most frequent. We encourage clinicians not only to evaluate the presence of these when working with ambivalent resistance, but also to address others that may be present in their clients.

We should also note that the discrepancies that we have observed are also not fixed or static. Work with self-discrepancies may evolve so that the selves that are relevant later in the work are different from the selves that began the discrepancy work. For example, in an initial two-chair assessment with a depressed client, the two selves that emerged were a Should Self and Reactant Self. The Should Self was clear about her need to work through her depression, while the Reactant Self made it clear that she didn't like being told what to do. Work with this client continued to use two two-chair dialogue method described in more detail in Chapters 6 and 7. In the next session, she renamed the selves "Be Close Self" and "Don't Be Close Self." These seemed more like a Should Self and a Fearful Self, respectively. In the following session, the two selves were identified as the "Giving Self" and the "Shy Self" (paralleling the Desired Self and the Fearful Self). As two-chair work proceeded, she returned to the Should Self and a less reactant and more positive self, which she named her "Positive Self." This kind of evolution is fairly characteristic of working with selves and discrepancies among them in two-chair work. The case is discussed in more detail in Chapter 10.

The integrative model presented in this chapter has a great deal in common with an approach called "motivational interviewing" (Miller & Rollnick, 1991, 2002) and gestalt two-chair therapy, both of which are discussed more fully in subsequent chapters. It also has elements of psychoanalytic, cognitive-behavioral, family systems, constructivist, and reactance theory approaches. However, our model is one that is open to new discoveries about the reasons people are ambivalent and resistant and the self-schemas and discrepancies that may relate to their resistance. It is more of a framework into which new information can enter than a fixed theory. Similarly, the methods of working with ambivalent resistance presented in this book are not fixed. We discuss those that we have employed that are consistent with our model. We hope that other ways of approaching ambivalent resistant consistent with this framework will also be found in the future.

SUMMARY

An integrated model of resistance was proposed in which resistance is seen as ambivalence. In this model, resistance occurs when the person expresses some desire to change, believes that the change will improve his or her life, believes that effective strategies are available, has adequate information about executing those strategies, but nonetheless does not employ them sufficiently for change. This experience is accompanied by negative affect.

Nine assumptions form the basis for our model of understanding and working with resistant ambivalence. We assume that when ambivalence occurs, it is important to understand the sources of the ambivalence and to work with the person to resolve it. Our view is in sharp contrast to that of those that see ambivalent resistance as an obstacle to be overcome so that the "real" treatment can occur.

We discussed three patterns of discrepancies or conflict among self-schemas that we frequently observe in resistant ambivalence. These were discrepancies between Desired and Should Selves, between Desired and Feared Selves, and between Should and Reactant Selves. We encourage the clinician to be open to whatever schemas and discrepancies might be present in their clients, and offer these as illustrations of some of the more common ones we have observed in our own work.

CHAPTER 4

Measurement and Assessment of Resistance and Ambivalence

Given the importance of the concepts of resistance and ambivalence, we have been struck by the relative paucity of empirical attempts to measure these constructs. We found several measures that were closely tied to a particular therapy theory and several others that cut across different approaches. With a few exceptions, however, most of these measures have not been widely evaluated in research. The measurement of ambivalence has received even less attention than the measurement of resistance. Because of this situation, our review draws not only from the therapy literature, but also from promising measures in social psychology that have not yet been studied in the clinical context. We conclude the chapter with clinical methods that we have found useful for assessing ambivalence but that have not yet been evaluated in research.

SELF-REPORT QUESTIONNAIRES

Client Resistance Scale

Mahalik (1994) developed a self-report measure called the "Client Resistance Scale" based on the premise that resistance in therapy is a consistent effort on the part of the individual to avoid painful affect. The five subscales seem to relate to a common construct of defensiveness. Mahalik (1994) also presented some preliminary data supporting this measure.

University of Rhode Island Change Assessment Scale

Prochaska and his associates developed the University of Rhode Island Change Assessment Scale (URICA), often referred to as the Stages of Change Questionnaire, based on their transtheoretical model (Prochaska & Norcross, 2004a). This model suggests that change involves progress through a series of five stages: precontemplation, contemplation, preparation, action, and maintenance. The URICA is designed to measure four of these stages. It consists of 32 items comprising four scales: precontemplation, contemplation, action, and maintenance. Each item is rated on a 5-point Likert scale of degree of agreement. Preparation is not included as a separate scale because the results of factor analyses suggested that it showed considerable overlap with the other stages. Prochaska and Norcross (2002) suggest that people who are in the preparation stage score high on both the contemplation and action scales. Subjects receive scores on each of the four scales. Change is assumed to be a continuous and oscillating process in which people move back and forth between stages. An individual can score high on more than one of the four scales. Individual stage scores can be determined by profiles using all four scales or by using the highest scale score.

The two stages most relevant to resistance and ambivalence are precontemplation and contemplation. According to Prochaska and Norcross (2004), precontemplation is the stage in which the individual does not intend to take action to change in the near future. People who score high on this scale appear to be unmotivated and resistant to change. Contemplation is the stage most closely associated with resistance and ambivalence about change. In this stage, the individual is aware that a problem exists and is seriously thinking about overcoming it in the near future, but has not yet made a commitment to do so. In this stage, the individual is more aware of the pros of changing, but is also struggling with the cons, such as the advantages of holding to the target behavior and the effort and energy required to change the target behavior. The balance between the costs and benefits of changing are believed to result in ambivalence.

Research on the URICA has been extensive (see reviews by Prochaska & Norcross, 2004a, 2004b). The scale has been used successfully to predict treatment outcome and dropouts in smoking treatment and other health-related behaviors. However, the transtheoretical model and the URICA have also been the target of numerous criticisms (e.g., Littel & Gurvin 2002; Sutton, 1996; Wilson & Schlam, 2004). For example, Littel and Gurvin (2002) concluded that, with the exception of the precontemplation state, the different stages of change have not been found to be discrete. They suggest that most participants do not fit neatly into one of the stages, and that subjects often endorse two items representing nonadjacent stages. Wilson and Schlam (2004) reviewed a number of studies on the URICA in predicting treatment outcome, and concluded that support for the URICA in this regard was mixed.

Most research on the URICA has concerned health-related behaviors rather than problems typically addressed in psychotherapy. While it may be a useful measure, more research must be conducted on the URICA in the area of psychotherapy and behavior change.

Selves Questionnaire

Since in our view ambivalence can be viewed as discrepancies among self-schemas, it is necessary that we have the tools to measure the relevant self-schemas, and also a way to measure the discrepancies among them that we believe may account for ambivalence. In this regard, we were fortunate to have available the work of such cognitive researchers as Higgins (1987, 1996) and Markus and Nurius (1986), who have provided some fascinating leads for the measurement of self-schemas that may relate to ambivalence and change. We should note, however, that these measures have been used primarily in research with college students.

The Selves Questionnaire, developed by E. Tory Higgins and his associates, has been used to measure self-schemas associated with different affective states (Higgins, 1987; Higgins, Klein, & Strauman, 1985). In our work, we have adapted the measure slightly to better fit clients in psychotherapy. Figure 4.1 presents the general instructions and a sample page from this questionnaire regarding the Desired Self, and Figure 4.2 gives the instructions for the other selves.

The questionnaire is an open-ended one that yields lists of adjectives or phrases that the person believes to be characteristic of his or her different self-schemas. Higgins, who has been interested in discrepancies between self-schemas, has developed a way of scoring these discrepancies (see Higgins, 1987, Higgins et al., 1985, for more detailed scoring information). However, these take considerable time and are probably more useful for research than practice. In the scoring, the first entry in one list (e.g., Desired Self) is compared to each entry in the second list

General Instructions: A particular aspect of your self-concept is described below (e.g., your "Actual Self," "Desired Self," etc.). List the characteristics you believe describe that aspect of your self-concept. You may use single words or brief phrases and you may list up to 10 characteristics for each. After you complete each page, please read over each characteristic you listed and rate each one on a 1–4 scale as described at the bottom of each page.

DESIRED SELF

Instructions: Below, please list the characteristics of the self that you DESIRE TO BE. When you list the characteristics, do not pay attention to the numbers following each line. After you have finished the listing, please read the instructions at the bottom of the page and go back and rate each characteristic.

CHARACTERISTICS OF THE SELF THAT I DESIRE TO BE

1. _____   1 2 3 4

2. _____   1 2 3 4

3. _____   1 2 3 4

4. _____   1 2 3 4

5. _____   1 2 3 4

6. _____   1 2 3 4

7. _____   1 2 3 4

8. _____   1 2 3 4

9. _____   1 2 3 4

10. _____ 1 2 3 4

Now, please go back to this list and rate each characteristic on the EXTENT TO WHICH YOU DESIRE TO HAVE THAT CHARACTERISTIC.

I desire to possess this characteristic:

1: Slightly   2: Somewhat   3: Moderately   4: Extremely

FIGURE 4.1. Selves Questionnaire for Desired Self. From Higgins, Klein, and Strauman (1985). Copyright 1985 by Springer Publishing. Adapted by permission.

Below, please list the characteristics of the self that you . . .
. . . actually consider yourself to be now. (Actual Self)
. . . should be. (Should Self)
. . . are afraid of becoming. (Feared Self)

FIGURE 4.2. Instructions for the other selves in the Selves Questionnaire. From Higgins, Klein, and Strauman (1985). Copyright 1985 by Springer Publishing. Adapted by permission.

(e.g., Should Self). A pair is considered to be a "match" if a thesaurus lists them as synonyms and their extent ratings differ by no more than 1 point. A "mismatch" is scored if they are listed as antonyms, and a "nonmatch" occurs when they are neither synonyms nor antonyms. Another category, and the most frequent type of mismatch, is "mismatch of degree," in which the words are synonyms, but differ by 2 or more extent points. In this way, each entry in the first list is compared to each entry in the second list. The results of such a comparison will yield a score for number of matches, number of mismatches, number of mismatches of degree, and number of nonmatches. One way that discrepancies have been quantified (Higgins, 1987; Higgins et al., 1985) is to take a ratio of the sum of the two types of mismatches over the sum of the matches. The larger the ratio, the greater the discrepancy.

For the comparison of the Desired Selves and the Should Selves, a low score on discrepancy suggests that what the person desires to be and what he or she believes he or she is are relatively congruent, and so there should be little ambivalence resulting from this comparison. By contrast, if the discrepancy score is relatively high, it suggests that what the person desires to be (e.g., laid back and relaxed) differs either in content or degree from what he or she believes he or she should be (e.g., hard-working and successful). This discrepancy is indicative of what Dollard and Miller (1950) called "a double approach–avoidance conflict." The more the person approaches one of the selves, the more uncomfortable he or she becomes because he or she is moving away from the other. This pattern would be suggestive of ambivalence.

By contrast, the comparison between Desired Selves and Feared Selves would indicate that less discrepancy (and more congruence) is suggestive of ambivalence. A low discrepancy score here suggests that the person both desires and fears the characteristics that were matches.

The more the person approaches those characteristics, the more fearful he or she becomes, leading to avoidance. The more he or she avoids, the more his or her desire for that characteristic leads to approach. An individual with social phobia who both desires to become more sociable and also intensely fears becoming more social is one example of this type of pattern.

Table 4.1 presents the responses of a depressed and anxious young woman to three of the selves in the Selves Questionnaire. The adjectives she used in the Actual Self reflect her mainly negative self-perceptions including "depressed," "insecure," and "fearful." Not surprisingly, the characteristics of her Desired Self are characteristic of someone who is neither depressed nor fearful. In comparing her Desired and Should Selves, we see signs of ambivalence. The Should Self gives a picture of an assertive, decisive, and successful woman driven by ambition. The Desired Self contains no such characteristics, but instead suggests a happy, funny, and compassionate person. The client came from a family of highly successful and wealthy professionals and she had certainly internalized "shoulds" that she should be like them. However, she was unsure if she wanted that life, or wanted a simpler life with a more modest career, family, and friends. After graduating from college, where she did quite well, she worked in a small business. She made sporadic attempts to explore admission to medical school, none of which went as far as actually submitting an application. Her ambivalence is reflected in the discrepancies between her Desired and her Should Selves.

The Reactant Self-schema involves a conflict between a self that gives a directive (often including a demand introduced by "You should . . . ") and another self-schema that reacts oppositionally. Measurement

TABLE 4.1. Selves Questionnaire Responses in a Case of Anxiety and Depression

Actual Self	Desired Self	Should Self
Depressed	Compassionate	Motivated
Curious	Funny	Ambitious
Insecure	Self-confident	Decisive
Fearful	Competent	Unafraid
Reserved	Happy	Optimistic
Sensitive	Supportive	Successful
Loyal		Assertive

of this interaction presents some unique problems. First, giving people instructions to list the characteristics of their Reactant Self is paradoxical. The more reactant they are, the less likely they should be to comply with our requests. We believe that other methods of measurement are necessary for measuring reactance; these are discussed later in the chapter.

Interrater reliability of measures derived from the Selves Questionnaire has been high because the scoring is relatively automatic based on a proper use of the thesaurus. however, there do not as yet exist norms for discrepancy scores, so they can only be used as a rough guide to ambivalence at the present time.

Van Hook and Higgins (1988) found that discrepancies between the Desired Self and the Should Self were associated with the affect of confusion, which may be a manifestation of ambivalence. Further, Arkowitz and Engle (1995) conducted a study with 14 people diagnosed with major depression. We found that subjects with high discrepancy scores at pretreatment did significantly poorer in therapy than subjects with low discrepancy scores. The discrepancy score at pretest correlated −.85 with changes in the main dependent variable, which was a composite depression score based on several well-validated inventories of depression. Discrepancy scores also decreased from pre- to posttreatment, as one might expect. Dropouts had much higher discrepancy scores at pretest than did the completers. Our initial attempts to relate these discrepancy scores to other indicators of resistance such as therapists' ratings, client lateness, and cancellations were not significant.

An interesting feature of the discrepancy method for measuring ambivalence is that the subject him- or herself does not have to be aware of discrepancies in order for us to measure them. People are asked to list the characteristics of each self. They are not asked about conflict, nor do they have any idea that we are interested in the relationships between entries in different lists. In this way, it may be possible to objectively measure conflicts and discrepancies without the subject having to be consciously aware of the conflict/discrepancy.

The Selves Questionnaire is a very promising direction for the measurement of ambivalence. Scoring requires the use of a thesaurus and can take 20–30 minutes. However, we have found that even without formal scoring, the Selves Questionnaire yields useful qualitative information on self-schemas and on ambivalence for clients in psychotherapy. We have also noted that clients have often found it a difficult and challenging test to take. It requires them to generate information that they don't usually think about—sometimes the results are surprising, even to the test taker. I (HA) once administered the Selves Questionnaire as an exercise to a graduate class in psychotherapy. While he was filling it out, one of the older students in the class uttered "Damn!" After class, he explained his behavior. He said that he'd been very ambitious and career-oriented most of his adult life, and didn't have much time for a social life. He noticed that his Should Self contained several words and phrases relating to ambition and success. However, he also noted that his Desired Self contained a number of responses that suggested his desire for a partner and a family. While he was somewhat aware of these desires, filling out the questionnaire helped him to crystallize them.

METHODS AND MEASURES
BASED ON DIRECT OBSERVATION

A number of published reports have used coding systems for resistance based on direct observation. Some have been based on ratings from observed behavior and others on coding systems for resistance.

Rating Measures

Psychoanalytic researchers have primarily emphasized rating measures of resistance and applied them to tapes or transcriptions of therapy sessions. The rating dimensions have been derived from psychoanalytic conceptualizations of resistance. Some examples include the work of Graff and Luborsky (1977), Luborsky et al. (1980), Morgan, Luborsky, Crits-Cristoph, Curtis, & Solomon, 1982). A good example of this work is a study by Schuller, Crits-Cristoph, and Connolly (1991). They developed a 19-item rating scale for evaluating the frequency and intensity of a variety of patient behaviors that are usually seen as indicative of resistance in psychoanalytic treatment. Scales generated from factor analysis revealed four dimensions of resistance: abrupt/shifting, oppositional, flat/halting, and vague/doubting. Reliabilities of the scales were acceptable but somewhat low, and the oppositional category was relatively infrequent.

Behavioral Measures

In two research programs using direct observation, coding systems have been developed for behaviors thought to indicate resistance. The first is in the work by Gerald Patterson and his associates (e.g., Chamberlain et al., 1984; Patterson & Chamberlain, 1994) on the training of parents of antisocial children in behavioral child management techniques. Their initial focus has been on the more obvious forms of resistance they encountered when working with these families. A scale with the following seven resistance categories was developed (Patterson & Chamberlain, 1994).

- Defend (Other or Self)
- Hopeless, Blame, Complain
- Challenge/Confront, Complain, Disagree
- Own Agenda, Sidetrack
- Answer For (Another)
- Intrafamily Conflict
- Disqualify (contradict One's Previous Statements)

They also coded "nonresistant statements" that included statements that were neutral, cooperative, or that followed the direction of the therapist. "Resistant statements" accounted for approximately 6% of the parents' utterances, and mostly consisted of "I can't" statements. Decreases in parents' resistant behaviors over the course of treatment was accompanied by more positive parenting behavior. In addition, parental resistance was associated with increased teaching and confrontation by the therapist, a greater number of sessions required for treatment, and a reduction in the therapist's liking for the client. By using a coding system that stays close to the observed data, some fascinating results emerged. Their work is noteworthy not only for its study of resistance in parent training, but as a method for studying resistance that might be employed in other areas of psychotherapy and change. As Patterson and Chamberlain (1994) correctly note, behaviors indicative of resistance in the parent training arena may be rather different from what constitutes resistance in other problem areas or types of therapy (e.g., individual cognitive or psychoanalytic therapy).

Miller, Benefield, and Tonigan (1993) adapted Patterson and Chamberlain's (1994) behavioral coding scale for resistance for coding interactions between alcoholics and their therapists. They found that alcoholics' consumption of alcohol 12 months later was predictable from resistant behaviors coded during the first treatment session 1 year earlier. These included interrupting; off-task responses such as inattention, silence, or side-tracking; and negative responses such as blaming others, disagreeing, and expressing reluctance or unwillingness to change.

While coding resistant behaviors from direct observation has yielded interesting results, the method is not very practical for the consulting room. In addition to generating research on resistance, these approaches may, however, aid the clinician to make informal observations of client behaviors possibly indicative of resistance.

MEASURING REACTANCE

Attempts to measure reactance have been based on either a state or a trait view. As a state, reactance is thought to be situation-specific. As a trait, it is thought to be a personal characteristic that manifests itself across situations.

Reactance as a State

Shoham-Salomon, Avner, and Neeman (1989) developed a measure of state reactance. They suggested that reactance is not amenable to direct questioning, since a subject would not openly admit to being reactive. In their study, reactance was inferred from the subjects' tone of voice. This was based on findings from literature on nonverbal communication that it is more difficult to control one's responses in nonverbal versus verbal channels (e.g., Zuckerman, DePaulo, & Rosenthal, 1986). Shoham-Salomon et al.'s method is unobtrusive, since subjects are unaware that it is their tone of voice that is being measured.

In their procedure, Shoham-Salomon et al. (1989) got tape-recorded responses from procrastinators to questions about the extent to which they can control and overcome their procrastination without outside help. They then altered the audio quality of the tape so that the actual words being said were undecipherable, but the subjects' tone of voice and speaking cadences could still be discerned; in other words, leaving the "music" of the speech without the "lyrics." These filtered recordings were coded on three intercorrelated dimensions (active–passive; spiteful–nonspiteful, and inhibited–uninhibited) to form a reactance score. Subjects were randomly assigned to one of two brief treatments: self-control (low reactance-evoking) or paradoxical treatment (high reactance-invoking). As predicted, subjects high on initial reactance benefited more from the paradoxical than from the self-control treatment. Also consistent with the predictions, there were no significant differences between high- and low-reactant subjects in the self-control condition. Shoham, Bootzin, Rohrbaugh, and Urry (1996) found a similar pattern of findings for insomnia patients given either paradoxical or skill-based interventions.

More recently, Davison and his associates have developed a novel method called "articulated thoughts in simulated situations" (ATSS; see review by Davison, Vogel, & Coffman, 1997). It has been used to measure state reactance in two studies (Gann, 1999; Gann & Davison, 1999), as well as anger–hostility (Davison, Williams, Nezami, Bice, & DeQuattro, 1991), irrational beliefs (Davison & Zighelboim, 1987), and cognitive bias in depression (White, Davison, Haaga, & White, 1992).

In the ATSS method, subjects listen to an audiotaped recording of actors in a simulated vignette, and are asked to imagine that they are in the situation as an observer. Each situation is divided into segments. After each segment, there is a free-response period in which the subjects are asked to verbalize their thoughts aloud. These thoughts are subsequently transcribed and coded. The stimulus situations and the coding system can both be varied to accommodate the constructs that the investigator wishes to study.

Using the ATSS method, Gann and Davison (1999) presented college students with situations in which they overheard interactions between a therapist and a client with an anxiety problem. In some situations, the therapist was using a defiance-based paradoxical therapy approach designed to elicit reactance. An example of one of these situations is:

Don't fight the anxiety, try to bring it on. This will give us a better chance to understand its nature by observing it while it happens. Every day, put yourself in as many anxious situations as possible and carefully observe and record every aspect of the anxiety as it intensifies. Do you think you can do that? [tone]

In other situations, the therapist worked from a behavioral approach not intended to elicit reactance. An example of this type of situation is:

I can teach you skills you can use to reduce your anxiety in these situations. But before we begin, we'll need to get more information about when your anxiety occurs. For the next week I want you to observe very carefully when you become anxious and what it feels like. What do you think? [tone]

Subjects' responses were coded for reactance on 5-point Likert scales ranging from "not defiant at all" to "totally defiant." As predicted, it was found that ATSS reactance scores, as indicated by defiant thoughts, were significantly greater for the paradoxical condition than for the behavioral condition. No relationship was found between ATTS state reactance scores and Dowd's self-report trait measure, the Therapeutic Reactance Scale (reviewed below). Gann (1999) replicated these findings with a clinical population of women with borderline personality disorder.

Both reactance measures described above are promising steps toward the measurement of the construct. In four studies, the validity of the state reactance measures was strongly supported. While both measures have been developed for use in research, they also have the potential for measuring reactance in clinical settings. At present, both are somewhat cumbersome for clinical use, requiring equipment and coding. In this regard, the ATSS might be easier to employ in clinical settings since the Shoham-Salomon et al. (1989) measure requires specialized voice filter equipment. If more user-friendly methods for measuring state reactance can be developed, the possibility of clinicians using them to assess reactance will be greatly enhanced.

Reactance as a Trait

One of the earliest attempts to measure reactance was the Therapeutic Reactance Scale (TRS) developed by Dowd, Milne, and Wise (1991). The TRS is a 28-item self-report questionnaire that includes such questions as "I resent authority figures who try to tell me what to do." In the original TRS, reliability was adequate. Significant negative correlations in the expected direction were obtained between the TRS and the K Scale of the MMPI as well as measures of locus of control. Dowd, Wallbrown, Sanders, and Yesehosky (1994) found correlations between the TRS and scales on the California Personality Inventory such as lack of interest in making a good impression on others, being less tolerant of others' beliefs, and resisting rules and regulations. However, Dowd et al.

(1988) did not find predicted differences between defiance-based and compliance-based treatment strategies for high- and low-reactant depressed patients. In a subsequent study, Swoboda, Dowd, and Wise (1990) found that level of reactance did not predict depressed patients' responses to either a reframing or a restraining intervention. More recently, in a well-controlled study high in statistical power, Arnow, Manber, and Blasey (2003) examined whether reactance, as measured by the TRS, would predict outcome in the treatment of depression. They did not find the predicted negative relationships between reactance and outcome. In fact, on two of four measures of outcome, the TRS was *positively* correlated with outcome.

Beutler and his associates (Beutler, Engle, et al., 1991; Beutler, Moleiro, & Talebi, 2002) have also developed a self-report measure related to trait reactance that they call "Resistance Potential" (RP). It is based on an arithmetic combination of MMPI scales of manifest anxiety and social defensiveness, with high scores presumably reflecting high resistance potential. Beutler, Engle, et al. (1991) predicted and found that high-RP depressed patients did better with a less directive treatment (self-directed therapy) and worse with more directive therapist-administered treatments, while the converse was true for low-RP depressed patients. These results were cross-validated at 1 year follow-up (Beutler, Machado, Engle, & Mohr, 1993) and replicated with a cross-cultural sample (Beutler, Mohr, Grawe, Engle, & McDonald, 1991).

A recent study by Baker, Sullivan, and Marszalek (2003) administered the TRS and the RP to a sample of depressed patients. They found that the two measures did not correlate despite their presumed ability to measure the same construct. In addition, the RP exhibited extremely poor internal consistency, calling into question results that have been based on this measure. Both of these self-report trait measures hold some promise, but considerably more research is necessary before we can feel confident that they do indeed measure the construct of reactance. However, as Shoham et al. (2004) have pointed out, it may be that we will make most progress by focusing our efforts on a state versus a trait measure of reactance. This makes good sense. If we want to know how reactant a person will be in a specific situation (e.g., in a particular type of therapy), then we should measure the characteristic of interest in a manner that stays close to that situation. In this regard, the state measures do much better than the trait measures. Further, while there is considerably less research on state measures of reactance, results have been consistent and supportive, while results for trait measures are considerably more mixed.

QUALITATIVE METHODS FOR ASSESSING RESISTANT AMBIVALENCE

In this section, we consider ways of qualitatively assessing resistant ambivalence that we have found clinically useful, but that have not yet been studied in research.

Markers of Ambivalence about Change

What are some of the indicators, or "markers," of ambivalence that we may detect in the course of a therapy session? Our discussion is in part based on the work of Greenberg et al. (1993) and their discussion of markers of what they call "conflict-split." We can usually see markers of ambivalence in the client's verbal behavior when he or she makes one statement that indicates a desire or need to change, and another that indicates a reluctance to do so or elaborates on the "costs" of changing. The two statements are in opposition, usually occur in close proximity to one another, and typically exhibit some sense of conflict or struggle. Some of the more common types of verbal statements that we consider to be markers of resistant ambivalence are:

- "On the one hand . . . , but on the other hand . . ."
- "Yes, but . . ."
- "Part of me wants to . . . , but part of me doesn't . . ."

Both types of statements reflect real positions of the person, but they stand in opposition to one another in the form of an approach–avoidance conflict. The more one side of the person tries to change, the more the other side pulls him or her back from these attempts; and the more the person pulls back from attempts to change, the more he or she is pulled toward trying to change. Some clinical examples of markers of ambivalence include remarks such as:

> "I know I should break up with him because he's no good for me, but I'm so afraid of being alone."

"On the one hand, I know that losing weight will be good for my health and make me feel better about myself, but on the other hand I'm not sure if I can do it."

"Yes, I know it would be good for me to speak up in meetings, but I feel afraid that what I have to say will be laughed at."

"I'm afraid that if I leave my wife, I'll be even unhappier than I am today."

"Yes, I know it would be good for my depression to become more active, but I just don't feel like it."

Another marker of ambivalence is a discrepancy between words and actions. For example, a depressed man may end a therapy session feeling more encouraged about overcoming his depression. He may tell the therapist that he plans to be more active and to get out of the house more in the coming week. Nevertheless, at the next session, the man reports that he couldn't get himself to be more active during the past week. His verbal statements point in one direction, while his behavior points in another. We believe that markers such as these contain the initial entry point for understanding and working with ambivalence about change. In the ensuing chapters, we outline how therapists can use such entry points for helping people resolve ambivalence and move toward change.

Two-Chair Assessment of Resistant Ambivalence

This method provides clinical data based on the client's performance during a modified two-chair procedure from gestalt therapy (Perls et al., 1951) or what has more recently been called "process–experiential therapy" (Greenberg et al., 1993). In the procedure, as we have adapted it, the client is first told that most people have some ambivalence about change, and that we would like to get to know these mixed feelings better. A focus for the change has usually been determined prior to the assessment (e.g., decreased depression, increased self-knowledge and insight, improvement in one's marital relationship).

To assess ambivalence with this clinical method, the therapist might talk to a client who treatment for depression in the following manner:

"Most people have mixed feelings about change, and I assume that you do as well. Part of the person really wants to change, but another part seems to struggle against the change. In your case, there may be a part of you that really wants to become less depressed, and another part of you that struggles against your attempts to get less depressed. Does that fit you at all? [If so, continue].

[Move an empty chair so that it faces the client.] "Let's start by having you be the side of you that really wants to be less depressed. Shortly, we'll sit the side of you that struggles against your attempts to change in that other chair. Speak in the first person to that other side in the empty chair, and tell it about yourself. For example, you might start by saying: 'I'm the side of Frank that really wants to get rid of my depression.' Continue from there to tell the other side what you think and feel about getting rid of your depression, always using 'I' and speaking in the first person."

After the client seems to have run out of things to say in this chair, ask him or her to switch chairs, and when he or she does, say something like "Now, be the side of yourself that struggles against changing your depression and doing the things you know would help, and speak to the other side from this perspective." In order to best use this approach, the interaction between the two sides should be extended. In subsequent chapters we discuss how to do this in more detail. At this point, we wish to highlight the following:

1. In this procedure, the role of the therapist is one of facilitator. Consistent with this role, the therapist does not interpret what is said or comment on it. The therapist primarily tries to facilitate the emerging interaction between the two sides.

2. The therapist should try to facilitate "contact" between the two sides. After one side has completed its "turn" and the client has changed seats to the other side, the therapist might say something like "Tell that side how what he (or she) just said makes you feel." For example, a depressed male client sitting in the "change" chair started to address the "struggle-against-change" chair in a bossy authoritarian way, telling him all the things he should do to correct his depression, such as exercise more, eat a proper diet, push himself to socialize more, and so on. After switching chairs and being asked to respond to the "change" chair with how he felt in the "struggle-against-change" chair, he responded angrily, indicating that he resented being told what to do without receiving any sympathy for how hard he was already trying. In our terms, what seemed to emerge was a conflict between a Should Self and a Reactant Self. As the interaction progressed, another "self" emerged in the "struggle-against-change" chair, which resembled a Feared Self that re-

sponded to the Should Self by saying that he was fearful that if he tried harder to do all of those things and failed, he'd feel even worse than he would if he didn't try at all.

Subsequent chapters discuss structuring and working with such two-chair interactions. Our point here is that the early phases of such interactions may provide useful clinical information about the various discrepant schemas involved in the client's ambivalence about change.

SUMMARY

There have been many attempts to measure resistance, but fewer to measure ambivalence. While there are many promising beginnings, and some qualitative methods that may be clinically useful, measurement of resistance and ambivalence needs a great deal more work. Two different self-report measures hold promise. The URICA measures stages of change, with the contemplation stage most closely associated with resistant ambivalence. The Selves Questionnaire comes closest to measuring ambivalence, and though it has been used in basic social psychological research, there have not as yet been any major clinical applications that have evaluated the measure.

Several measures have been developed that involve rating or coding client behavior during therapy sessions. These have proven useful in research but are cumbersome for clinical use, requiring transcription of the sessions and labor-intensive coding. Measures of reactance both as a state and as a trait have been developed, but the trait measures have been self-report inventories. As such they are more convenient for clinical use and have not performed so well in the research that's evaluated them. The two kinds of measures of state reactance we described that employ (1) filtered voice or (2) a think-aloud approach (the ATSS) are also promising, but, once again, they require somewhat elaborate equipment in the former case and coding in both cases, making them inconvenient for clinical applications. We concluded with a discussion of qualitative methods that we have found clinically useful for assessing ambivalence. One involved attention to markers of resistance during the session and the other a modified two-chair assessment procedure designed to target ambivalence about change.

CHAPTER 5

An Overview of Approaches to Working with Resistant Ambivalence

We have proposed a model in which resistant ambivalence is a core experience in psychotherapy, health care, and self-change. We have suggested that helping people to resolve this ambivalence leads to better therapeutic outcomes. In the remainder of this book, we discuss therapeutic approaches to deal with resistant ambivalence that are consistent with our framework.

We searched the literature widely for ways of working with ambivalence consistent with our approach. We found many publications that were relevant, but the authors of these papers seemed to be unaware of others who thought similarly. These therapy strategies were often based on rather different theoretical rationales and involved different therapy operations. So we have tried to bring them all together under one framework.

Some of these approaches, like two-chair work and motivational interviewing, were more highly developed clinically and more extensively researched than others. Because of this, we devote separate chapters to these two methods of working with resistant ambivalence. We also discovered other approaches that were not specifically designed to resolve resistant ambivalence, although they can be used for that purpose by inference. These approaches also have little or no research associated with them. They are reviewed in this chapter.

These approaches are all based on a strong partnership between the client and the therapist and involve an accepting stance by the therapist. The therapist adopts a curious and exploratory attitude and tries to understand the client's experience. This accepting attitude has several implications. First, that the therapist views all data as informative and friendly. The failure of a client to change, to complete homework assignments, and so on is informative and suggests ambivalence, but not obstinate resistance. Second, therapists working from this perspective do not advocate for any particular outcome. They listen for all the voices of the client's experiences and patiently invite each voice into full awareness where it can be more completely explored and understood. Third, therapists using these approaches realize that the client may not be fully aware of the presence of or nature of his or her discrepant schemas. Often the client only knows that he or she sincerely desires to change and is not succeeding at making change. Fourth, the therapist works with the client to help resolve differences and discrepancies among the various schemas.

VOICE DIALOGUE

Stone and Stone (1989, 1991; Stone & Winkelman, 1985) describe their approach as "voice dialogue." While they originally came from the Jungian tradition, they broke away from it to found their own approach. They view voice dialogue as compatible with most psychological systems. Their approach is not oriented toward psychopathology but toward an exploration of the multiple voices *as they are* in a person rather than as what they *should be*. Each voice is different and is explored as fully as possible. The therapeutic goal is for the client to accept opposing viewpoints and to make decisions that take them into account. Even though they don't discuss how their model applies to resistance or ambivalence, we believe it has potential in this regard.

Stone and Stone postulate that accommodation to opposing viewpoints is accomplished by the "Aware Ego" that is understood to be a separate from any of the selves. They offer a specific technique for working with different voices or subpersonalities. The method is fairly well delineated (Stone & Stone, 1989, 1991). In the first step, the therapist/facilitator settles into a relaxed yet alert state. In the second step, the therapist creates a "psychic map." The therapist listens carefully to a description of a troubling issue in the subject's life. The therapist begins to identify primary selves and the opposite characteristics that are disowned. Some selves emerge often enough that the facilitator may watch for them: the Protector/Controller, the Pusher, the Critic, the Perfectionist, the Power Broker, the Pleaser, the Inner Child, the Good and Bad Mother/Father (1991, pp. 91–92). This list is not exhaustive and the client may exhibit other "disowned selves" such as the selfish, the comical, or the lazy self. *Disowned selves* are those selves that we do not wholly acknowledge or do not want to legitimize. For example, few want to admit to being uncaring and selfish in interactions with others.

In the third step, the therapist introduces the idea of different selves and elicits the client's responses to them. The experiment begins when the client reports that the facilitator has a correct understanding of his or her experience and is willing to pursue an exploration of these selves in a dialogue between a specific self and the therapist. In the fourth step, the therapist asks the client to move from his or her seat, reserved for the "Aware Ego," and to sit in another seat. This change in space serves to separate the selves. The selves may assume different positions in the room: for example, a vulnerable-child self may curl up on the couch, while a critical self may prefer to stand, and an angry self may pace.

The fifth step is the facilitation. When a self takes a new place in the room, the therapist begins to interact with that self as if it were a real and distinct person. At this point the facilitator uses all available clinical skills to interview the chosen self. The facilitation begins by exploring a self that has been identified as a primary self, leaving disowned selves to be explored in later sessions. Stone and Stone propose that primary selves are a rich source of information about the difficulties and dangers in the client's life. Selves usually speak to the therapist easily and freely unless the Protective Self takes over. If this occurs, the therapist and the client discuss the presence of the Protective Self and decide whether or not to continue the dialogue with one of the voices. In voice dialogue, the therapist works to recognize when one self gives way to another, and then proceeds to clarify the differences among the selves. Stone and Stone suggest that clients may be in a vulnerable state during this work because the individual voice is temporarily separate from the Aware Ego. Therefore, the therapist always returns the client to a primary self before he or she leaves the session, and always reinvolves the Aware Ego.

In the final steps of this procedure, the therapist and the client stand alongside each other as the therapist summarizes the major points of the session. Stone and Stone suggest that this method develops awareness in the client akin to that of a nonjudgmental observer who can see the selves, their roles, and their interactions. Finally the client is returned to the original chair reserved for the Aware Ego. This allows the client to separate from the selves that have spoken and to integrate the work of the session.

Applications to Resistance and Ambivalence

Although Stone and Stone do not specifically discuss this issue, we believe that voice dialogue has potential as a method of helping people to resolve their ambivalence. The method bears many similarities to the two-chair procedure discussed in Chapters 6 and 7. However, the therapist plays a more active role in voice dialogue. When the client does not change, the voice dialogue therapist could interview the self that wants to change while allowing the unchanging self to listen. Then the roles could be reversed, with the therapist interviewing the unchanging self. By interviewing the selves separately, as if they were two separate people driven by different sets of experiences, wants, and needs, ambivalence is explored as something natural. Such an exploration can potentially lead to a negotiated settlement of the ambivalence. Interviewing one self at a time allows the other self to listen to new information.

Evaluation

The voice dialogue approach is easily integrated into other therapies. The strategy is straightforward and relatively easy to use. However, it currently lacks any research evaluating its effectiveness. Nonetheless, we believe that this approach does have real potential and warrants further attention in both research and practice.

GESTALT APPROACHES

Gestalt practitioners, while grounded in common assumptions, vary widely in how they conduct therapy. We briefly present the approaches of three different gestalt therapists: Erving Polster (1995), Joseph Zinker (1977), and James Kepner (1987).

Polster

Polster (1995) takes the position that every person is a "population of selves." He categorizes selves into *essential selves* that are extremely enduring and *member selves* that are more in flux and often overshadowed. The goal of Polster's approach is to bring all member selves into the awareness of the client and to create a climate where different selves will each have a voice.

Zinker

Zinker (1977), also from the gestalt tradition, approaches selves as a collection of polarities. He believes that all people have a strong tendency to disown their unacceptable selves. Zinker asserts that a person cannot fully own one part of the self unless he or she fully embraces the polar opposite—for example, a person cannot fully express kindness unless he or she also embraces his or her hard, tough, unkind self. If the client presents as mean and self-critical, Zinker will ask the client to explore the polar opposite, the part that can love and nurture the self. Often this is done through the use of the two-chair enactment that has been a standard intervention in gestalt therapy since the time of Perls, Hefferline, and Goodman (1951). It is a logical extension to use this approach when people are ambivalent and manifest polar opposites of a self that seeks change and a self that seeks the status quo.

Kepner

Gestalt therapy has always attended to the physical components of the client's experience, such as body posture, voice tone, and breathing. Kepner (1987) believes that the body and its manifestations are as intrinsic to the self as mental functioning, and he chooses to work very directly with the body in the context of gestalt therapy. Kepner believes that gestalt therapy gives equal importance to both the body and mental functioning.

Both Kepner and Zinker use the cycle of gestalt formation and completion to inform their work. A healthy person interacts with the environment to meet his or her needs by moving smoothly through the gestalt cycle of sensation, figure formation, mobilization, action, contact, and withdrawal (as described in Chapter 2).

Clinical Applications

Although Polster's approach is grounded in gestalt therapy and the use of in-session experiments, such as "empty-chair" or "two-chair" experiments, they are not at the heart of his work. He proposes three ways to approach the population of selves: dialogue, accentuation, and orientation.

1. *Dialogue*. This is not a two-chair dialogue, but one that takes place between the therapist and the client. The therapist may become aware of the presence of different selves before the client does. When this occurs, the therapist names the different selves for the client and then elicits from the client the story behind each of the selves—drawing out all the struggles, hopes, and dreams of each self. This, in effect, breathes new life into the isolated selves. By learning about the isolation of the different selves, the client becomes aware of different personal characteristics that vie for recognition and ascendancy. Polster sometimes asks the client to engage in a dialogue between two selves (two-chair work), but he is concerned that excessive experimental dialogues like this may interfere with the necessary conversational engagement between the client and the therapist. He also fears that gestalt therapy is sometimes reduced to a set of gimmicky experiments.

2. *Accentuation*. The naming of selves by the client helps accentuate characteristics and experiences that otherwise might go unnoticed. Assigning a name for a particular set of characteristics (i.e., a self) adds a personal stake with which the client identifies more strongly. The client will benefit from naming and more fully understanding the different selves that occur in his or her life experience.

3. *Orientation*. Polster (1995) suggests that naming different selves increases the therapist's understanding of the client, providing guidance in the therapeutic interaction. The therapist tries to fully explore and understand all the selves.

Both Zinker and Kepner work with "resistance to contact" based upon where in the gestalt cycle the client is struggling. While Zinker's approach follows a more traditional gestalt therapy path, Kepner's interventions are, in large part, designed to work directly with the body. Interventions are based upon an understanding of where the client has problems in moving through the gestalt cycle.

Applications to Resistance and Ambivalence

In Polster's approach, people change not by changing an essential self, but by bringing another self into the community of selves. This is consistent with our view that in resistant ambivalence, the self that resists change needs to be brought to the table and made a part of the community of selves or voices.

For Zinker, the more a person fully engages the polar selves (e.g., peaceful vs. anxious) the more the person comes to accept how he or she is. It is the acceptance of the way things are that leads to the resolution of the tension that creates ambivalence. Paradoxically, the acceptance leads to change.

Kepner's work reminds us that ambivalence will have an effect on our bodies as well as on our minds and emotions. Even if a therapist does not choose to work directly with the client's body, Kepner's model offers a map by which a therapist can understand how to identify the nature of the ambivalence—by knowing where in the gestalt cycle the person is stuck. The body is an additional source of information about the resistant ambivalence. Based on Kepner's approach, we believe that ambivalence can occur at any transition in the gestalt cycle when the client resists contact with the next phase of the cycle. For example, in the transition from mobilization to action, there seems to be a self that naturally seeks to move into action and a self that resists taking action. We believe that the "resistances to contact" could be viewed as examples of resistant ambivalence.

Evaluation

The approaches of Polster and Kepner do not lend themselves to simple interventions that are easily incorporated into other therapy approaches. But Zinker's use of two-chair work is a well-defined strategy that can be readily adopted and adapted to work with resistant ambivalence. All three authors view resistance as an expression of a creative energy within the person that has been disowned, but is clamoring for recognition. We believe that the resolution of ambivalence is facilitated by such an attitude. Both Polster and Zinker describe a multitude of client "voices" or "selves," but neither has refined their interventions to specifically address ambivalence. Their formulations are consistent with our view of ambivalence as discrepancies among selves or voices. Nonetheless, there has not yet been any research examining either process or outcome in these three approaches.

PSYCHODRAMA

In psychodrama, clients *enact* events in their lives rather than *talk* about them. This kind of therapy is usually conducted in a group setting. Group members take an active role in the drama of others under the guidance of a trained practitioner known as the "director." An episode in a client's life is reenacted in a supportive setting that invites improvisational dramatic action. Group members participate in the spontaneous drama as significant others or as a "double" (stand-in) for the client who is working on a personal problem. The purpose of psychodrama is to allow clients to generate and practice new behaviors and test them out on those around them (other group members) before engaging in the new behaviors in day-to-day life.

Psychodrama does not work directly with the concept of resistance. If, in the course of engaging in the psychodrama, the client does not change, it is understood as a failure on the part of the therapist to properly "warm up" the client before the psychodrama begins (D. Baumgartner, personal communication, 2002). The task of psychodrama is to raise the spontaneity and creativity of the client sufficiently so that he or she begins to take on new roles. The therapist must create a safe place that reduces the client's fear of making mistakes. Psychodrama utilizes warm-up exercises to put the client at ease and to encourage openness to exploration. Blatner (1991, 1995) sees psychodrama as an adjunct to therapy rather than as a complete therapy in itself. He suggests that the techniques of psychodrama's can be used in individual, family, and group psychotherapies. The physical involvement in a psychodrama fosters a vivid, immediate experience that leads to emotionally based insight.

TECHNIQUES

Psychodrama has developed a multitude of techniques, and only a few of the more basic ones will be addressed here. One involves working with the emergence of different selves, that is, different psychological components of the psyche. In psychodrama, these selves engage in a dialogue that encourages each to speak without interruption so as to avoid any confusion. The Psychodrama leader and group interact with each self until that self has been thoroughly engaged and understood.

Another important technique is called "doubling" in which another group member takes a position next to the protagonist (client), and expresses their hunches about what may be the person's most inner (but unspoken) thoughts and feelings. Each active, empathic statement is checked carefully with the protagonist for accuracy. The use of doubling has the potential to bring another self into awareness where it can participate in the action-oriented therapy and become a more integrated part of the whole person.

Application to Client Ambivalence

Although Psychodrama doesn't directly deal with resistance or ambivalence, we can extrapolate from it to ways that it might be used for this purpose. Assume that a client (Psychodrama protagonist) is prepared for the Psychodrama and ready to try on new, spontaneous behaviors. The client may become "stuck" and have difficulty experimenting with new behaviors. This person may be in a state of ambivalence about change. One of several Psychodramatic interventions may be useful. This is a time when it may be helpful to invite some other member of the group to "double" for the client and give a voice to the self that is hesitant about engaging in the new behaviors. This voice may make explicit what has implicitly kept the client from changing. The success of this strategy depends upon the alertness and sensitivity of the "double" and upon an ongoing confirmation that what is spoken by the "double" is seen by the client as accurate.

It is also possible to ask someone from the group to assume the role of the "stuck self" that is hesitant to change. This person could engage in a dialogue with the client who desires change. Again, the success of this experiment depends on the ability of the role-player to capture the essence of the "stuck" self. Finally, we believe that ambivalence can be explored in Psychodrama by asking the client to play out both parts of the ambivalence sequentially and in dialogue with the facilitator or group members.

Evaluation

In the early part of the 20th century, Psychodrama had a strong impact on the field of group psychotherapy. However, there has been a decline in that influence which critics often credit to the paucity of empirical research (D'Amato & Dean, 1988). In the past 23 years, 4 reviews of outcome research on psychodrama found some promising results, but overall the data were insufficient and lacked sound methodologies (Kipper & Richie, 2003).

Perhaps the best evidence of empirical support appears in the meta-analysis conducted by Kipper & Richie (2003). These authors sought to determine the effect sizes of four different techniques—role-playing, role reversal, doubling and multiple techniques. They found 25 studies spanning the last 3 decades that met inclusion criteria of experimental designs and control groups. Role reversal and Doubling showed the largest improvements. Multiple techniques produced only moderate improvement and role-playing showed hardly any improvement.

SOLUTION-FOCUSED COUNSELING

Solution-Focused Counseling (SFC) came into being as a reaction to a problem-solving model that emphasized an understanding of *how* or *why* problems persist. SFC offers a "nonpathological" strengths or competency-based approach. SFC practitioners have confidence in the client's ability to make changes, and the therapy focuses on using those inner resources and strengths. The client directs the therapeutic process by voicing preferences and by determining the treatment goals (Berg & Miller, 1992; de Shazer, 1990; Walter & Peller, 2000).

SFC is based on several assumptions (Lewis & Osborn, 2004):

1. Change happens when therapy moves directly to the construction of solutions and does not dwell on the development of the problem. Practitioners believe that knowing a lot about a problem is not necessarily related to formulating a solution. Small changes in one area can lead to greater changes in other areas (the "ripple effect").

2. The counselor–client relationship is critically important. The counselor assumes the role of student and the client is viewed as the teacher. Clients are trusted to know and make decisions about what is best for them. There is an abiding curiosity about the client's abilities, strengths, and competencies.

3. Positive change is not a static event, but an action-based, process-oriented phenomenon. Action is the process through which changes in thinking and behavior take place.

4. SFC assumes that clients hold critical beliefs about how change related to their goals will happen. Counselors need to cooperate with these views (e.g., by using the same language as the client), while also facilitating the consideration of new possibilities.

Clinical Applications

SFC is not so much a therapy model as it is a philosophy about how to strengthen client motivation (Lewis & Osborn, 2004). In SFC, the therapist assumes that change is possible and is preoccupied with the discovery of "nonproblem occasions." For example, the therapist pursues those times during which a client encountered a difficult situation and managed to deal with it effectively, or when the client was able to "take a vacation" from the problem. These interventions are designed to move the focus away from the problem itself and toward creating solutions.

Two principles guide work with clients: (1) pacing—matching the client's tone, affect, and words to demonstrate an understanding and acceptance; and (2) inviting—using questions that gently explore new meanings or possibilities. These processes invite the client to construct a new reality. The SFC counselor assumes a "not-knowing" stance and engages in "wondering out loud" what might be helpful. The counselor and the client pursue a mutual, deliberate reflection about how to resolve the situation. While SFC recognizes that clients are often ambivalent, ambivalence is not a key focus of the therapy.

Lewis and Osborn (2004) suggest that SFC, although a "brief therapy," can be used appropriately as a more extended therapy as well. These authors also suggest that there can be a strong confluence between SFC and motivational interviewing (described later in this chapter and in Chapter 8). They believe that, in tandem, the two approaches create a strong therapeutic intervention. Practitioners of SFC avoid the term "resistance" and dispute the belief that people do not want to change. If a client does not follow the therapist's suggestion, that behavior is viewed as a sign that they are not on the same page (O'Hanlon & Weiner-Davis, 1989). Rather than break down resistance, the SFC therapist seeks to understand the client's idiosyncratic way of cooperating. The therapist makes every effort to interact with the client consistent with the client's worldview. SFC suggests that too often the term "resistance" is used when an impasse has been reached.

Applications to Resistance and Ambivalence

SFC therapists recognize that there is ambivalence in people who seek change (O'Hanlon, 2003). For example, O'Hanlon (2003) uses permissive language that allows the client to experience both sides of the ambivalence. In a sense, the therapist gives the client permission to either feel angry or to feel not angry, to be close or to be distant. For the most part, SFC therapists work with resistant ambivalence indirectly by assuming that it will fade if the client begins to focus on solutions.

Evaluation

The relative lack of research on SFC leaves us unable to draw any clear conclusions about its effectiveness. Many reports of successful outcome are based primarily on anecdotal evidence or on subjective clinical experience (Miller, 1994). Studies conducted by the Brief Family Therapy Center lacked solid methodology and were never published (Lewis & Osborn, 2004). Gingerich and Eisengart (2000) reviewed 15 SFC outcome studies and found only five that met established research criteria. Only two of those five reported significant outcomes.

COMMENTS

The approaches described above have potential for conceptualizing and working with resistant ambivalence. While we believe that they are worthy of further development and clinical experimentation, they also need to be subjected to closer research scrutiny. Some of these approaches (e.g., psychodrama in groups) would be difficult to integrate into other psychotherapy approaches. However, we do believe that they can be taken as a starting point for innovation by clinicians in dealing with resistant ambivalence.

The above approaches are limited by the fact that they were not originally designed to work with resistant ambivalence, but we argue that they can be extended for this purpose. In addition, they are limited by a lack of solid research support. By contrast, there are two other approaches that we believe are uniquely well suited for working with resistant ambivalence: the two-chair approach and motivational interviewing. Both are well-developed clinically, and both have generated either some (the two-chair approach) or a great deal (motivational interviewing) of research support. Both have great potential as a stand-alone treatment and as an approach that can be combined or integrated into other therapies. Below, we describe each of them briefly, but we will expand on both of these approaches in the next few chapters.

THE TWO-CHAIR APPROACH

Description

The two-chair approach has its roots in the gestalt therapy of Perls et al. (1951). These authors described the concepts of "top dog" and "underdog" (separate selves) and the use of experiments that encourage the client to create a dialogue between selves. In recent years, Leslie Greenberg and his associates have refined this strategy and added a strong humanistic, client-centered foundation (Greenberg & Safran, 1987; Greenberg et al., 1993). They described several splits or discrepancies between selves. The one of most relevance to ambivalence is what they call "conflict splits." Here, there is a sense of struggle between the two selves that pull a person in different directions. Based on the work of Greenberg et al. (1993), we developed the marker of ambivalence described earlier and a two-chair clinical method that can be used when such markers are observed.

The two-chair intervention creates an in-session dialogue between the discrepant selves relating to change. In our version of the conflict split, one self advocates *for* change and another self struggles *against* change. The dialogue is structured in an experiment in which the client speaks consecutively from two chairs that are placed facing one another. One self (the Change Self) speaks from one chair and the other self (the No Change Self) speaks from the other. The two-chair method is consistent with the assumptions about resistant ambivalence we discussed in Chapter 3. In addition, we want to emphasize the following points:

- The schematic contents of the self that resists change are often outside of awareness. Once the schema is brought to light through the two-chair process, it can be reshaped in a manner that is more useful for the individual and more conducive to his or her change.
- The two-chair method is a collaborative effort between the client and the therapist. The therapist accepts the worldview of the client and works from that perspective. The client is understood to be

the expert concerning his or her own experience. The "accepting" spirit of this approach is at least as important as the specific techniques.

- In the two-chair intervention, the therapist acts as a facilitator, keeping the client focused on present-moment experience, assisting the client in differentiating the different voices or selves that are at work, and promoting a meaningful dialogue between the separate selves. The therapist does not "side" with either of the voices.

- Two-chair work leads to an awareness and understanding of both sides of the ambivalence about change. Armed with a new awareness and understanding of the nature of the ambivalence, the client is more likely to arrive at a resolution of his or her ambivalent state.

- An increase of the client's emotional arousal during the two-chair dialogue is important because the aroused state facilitates access to underlying schematic material.

- The two-chair intervention can be used as a stand-alone approach or it can be integrated into other therapies.

Chapters 6 and 7 describe this intervention in more depth. Here, we consider research on the two-chair approach.

Research on the Efficacy of the Two-Chair Approach

Most of this research has been done by Leslie Greenberg and his associates. For the most part, these studies have examined relationships between process variables and outcome, and were not studies of the efficacy of the approach.

In one of the earliest studies on the two-chair procedure, Greenberg and Clarke (1979) compared two sessions of empathic reflection (derived from Carl Rogers's client-centered therapy [1951]) with two sessions of two-chair work for counseling psychology graduate students who were experiencing ambivalence about a decision. Subjects in the two-chair group showed a greater depth of experiencing and a greater shift in awareness than did subjects in the empathic reflection group. While both showed considerable movement toward goals, they were not significantly different from one another. In a follow-up study, Greenberg and Higgins (1980) again found greater depth of experiencing for the two-chair group compared to the empathic reflection group. However, there were no significant differences between these two groups on shifting awareness and progress toward goals, with both showing greater improvements on these measures than a no-treatment control group.

Greenberg and Dompierre (1981) studied clients in ongoing counseling who were given two experimental sessions during their course of treatment. In one session they were given two-chair work and in the other empathic reflection. There was a greater shift in awareness and depth of experience for subjects in the two-chair condition, but there were no differences between the two treatment groups in behavior change. Both groups did better on these measures than a control condition.

In another study using volunteers who were having trouble making a difficult decision, Greenberg and Webster (1982) gave all subjects a 6-week treatment consisting mainly of two-chair work. After the treatment, subjects were divided into "resolvers" and "non-resolvers" based on whether they had manifested three components of a proposed model of conflict resolution during treatment: expression of criticism by one side; expression of feelings and wants by the other; and a "softening" in the attitude of the critic. After treatment, resolvers were significantly less indecisive and anxious after treatment than non-resolvers.

Clarke and Greenberg (1986) employed subjects who sought counseling to help them resolve a conflictual decision. They were randomly assigned to two sessions of either a two-chair intervention or a problem-solving cognitive-behavioral intervention (CBT), or to a no-treatment control group. The two-chair group improved more than the CBT group and the control group on one measure of indecisiveness. The two groups did not differ significantly on the other measure; however, both groups improved significantly more than the no-treatment control group. Unfortunately, this study did not include any measures of behavior change.

More recently, Greenberg and Watson (1998) conducted a study of patients who met the criteria for major depression. They compared 15–20 sessions of either client-centered therapy (CCT) or process-experiential therapy (PET). The PET therapy included a base of CCT in the context of which the therapist used several different gestalt techniques including, but not limited to, two-chair dialogues for conflict splits. Overall, both groups showed considerable improvement with treatment. The effects seemed clinically significant when compared to effect sizes in other treatment studies of depression that employed a no-treatment control group. At posttreatment, the PET group showed greater improvements in self-esteem, interpersonal functioning, and symptom distress than did the CCT group. Further, PET seemed to work faster, showing greater changes than CCT at midtreatment. While treatment gains were maintained at 6-month follow-up, differences between the two treatments disappeared.

Arkowitz and Engle (1995) conducted a small pilot study on the two-chair procedure for resolving ambivalence. People who were having trouble making an important change in their lives were recruited by placing advertisements in the campus newspaper. Seven respondents were deemed appropriate for the study. The subjects included two women who wanted to leave what they considered to be bad relationships but were unable to do so, one smoker who wished to stop, one man who was trying to lose weight, one woman who was messy to the point of embarrassment about having people visit her, one woman who was indecisive in her career choice, and one depressed man who was unable to move ahead on many of the goals he had set for himself.

Engle and Arkowitz were both present and active in the therapy sessions. Each subject received four half-hour sessions devoted almost entirely to the two-chair procedure applied to the focal problem. We started with an assessment in which we asked the client to have a dialogue between the side that wants to change and the side that struggles against the change. We continued the dialogue for most of the session, as described in Chapters 6 and 7. Some distress measures were taken (e.g., the Brief Symptom Inventory) and we also evaluated progress toward their change goals. Of the seven, there were clear resolutions and behavioral changes in four, improvement short of full resolution and change in two, and no change at all in one. These results are based both on our posttreatment and 1-year follow-up interviews and measures.

The findings described in this section suggest that the two-chair procedure may be useful clinically, but the research base is too limited to draw any strong conclusions about efficacy. Most of the studies were not randomized clinical trials with patients, but rather were studies of process–outcome relationships, often with analogue populations volunteering for a research project or small samples. The one study that did use a carefully screened clinical population (Greenberg & Watson, 1998) compared two treatments but did not have a no-treatment control group. While results are promising, the jury is still out on whether the two-chair strategy is efficacious.

MOTIVATIONAL INTERVIEWING

Description

Motivational interviewing (MI), first described by Miller (1983), began as a way of working with the problems of alcohol and substance abuse, but more recently has expanded to other problems like anxiety and depression (Arkowitz & Westra, 2004). Miller and Rollnick (1991, 2002) have presented the background and methods in two books.

Miller and Rollnick (2002) describe MI as a client-centered *and* directive approach. It is client-centered in its basic humanistic underpinnings concerning how people and change are viewed. It also draws heavily from client-centered therapy including its emphases on reflection and empathy. It is directive only in a subtle sense. MI does not try to directly influence people to change. In fact, any therapist who adopts the stance of "change advocate" is not doing MI. Instead, the MI therapist seeks to increase intrinsic motivation and reduce ambivalence about changing. With these changes, it is assumed that behavior change will naturally occur, with the client perceiving that the locus of change is in him or her rather than in the therapist.

MI, like the two-chair approach, is entirely compatible with the integrative model of resistance that we have proposed. The two points of view share basic humanistic assumptions about human nature and the importance of client agency in change. They both also place great emphasis on ambivalence rather than resistance in understanding why people don't change. MI also offers well-developed and well-researched methods of working with ambivalence. For these reasons, we have devoted two chapters (Chapters 8 and 9) to it.

RESEARCH ON THE EFFICACY OF MI

Two comprehensive reviews of the efficacy of MI have recently appeared (Burke, Arkowitz, & Dunn, 2002; Burke, Arkowitz, & Menchola, 2003). The first of these is a qualitative review while the second is a meta-analysis. This section will draw from both of these reviews.

Burke et al. (2003) noted a rather odd phenomenon in the literature on MI: not one of the published treatment studies represented a "pure" case of the use of MI. Virtually all of the published studies describe research in which other components have been added to the basic MI procedures. Given this, it cannot be determined whether effects are due to the MI or to the added elements or to both. In many cases, the added element consisted of feedback to the client about his or her behavior. For example, all of the studies on alcoholism include a feedback procedure in which the client is informed about how his or her current drinking compares to drinking norms in our society. In other cases, non–MI techniques were added (e.g., some CBT techniques) to the MI. Since none of these can be considered as "pure" MI, the authors decided to label the MI-related procedures as adaptations of MI (AMIs).

The meta-analysis of Burke et al. (2003) reviewed 30 studies of AMIs applied as a prelude to other treatment or as a stand-alone treatment for problems including alcohol abuse, drug abuse, smoking, diet and exercise, and HIV-risk behaviors. They found that overall, when AMIs were compared to no-treatment or placebo controls, they did significantly better and yielded moderate effect sizes (from 0.25 to 0.57) for these comparisons. Further, AMIs were as effective as other treatments to which they have been compared.

There is some evidence from a large multisite alcohol treatment outcome study suggesting that AMIs may work faster than alternative treatments. With a sample size of 1,800 people with problem drinking, Project MATCH (Project MATCH Research Group, 1997) randomly assigned subjects to one of three treatments: a four-session AMI treatment, a 16-session CBT, or a 16-session 12-step treatment. All three treatments did well at posttreatment and 15-month follow-up, with only a few minor differences among them. The fact that a brief AMI did as well as much longer established treatments suggests the possibility that it works in a shorter period of time. However, the proper experiment for this conclusion has not been done. It would be instructive to compare four sessions of each of the treatments before we can draw any such conclusion.

In the Burke et al. (2003) meta-analysis, outcomes for AMIs were also examined separately for each main problem area. Results supported the efficacy of AMIs compared to no treatment or placebos for problems involving alcohol, drugs, and diet and exercise. For example, in the area of excessive drinking, AMIs showed 51% improvement rates, a 56% reduction in drinking behaviors, and effects on other drinking-related behaviors as well (e.g., driving under the influence of alcohol violations). Burke et al. (2003) reported effect sizes for drinking to range from 0.25 to 0.47 depending on the outcome measures employed. The effect size for drug use was 0.56 and the effect size for diet and exercise was 0.53. Results did not support the efficacy of AMIs for smoking and HIV-risk behaviors, although it should be noted that the number of studies in each of the latter categories was quite small. Finally, in those studies of AMIs that included follow-ups, the effects of AMIs maintained well over time for the follow-up periods that were reported (up to about a year).

AMIs as a Prelude to Treatment

As we discuss in more detail in Chapter 10, there is strong research support for the use of AMIs as a prelude to subsequent treatment. The meta-analysis by Burke et al. (2003) included 14 studies of AMIs as a prelude and found strong support for the effectiveness of such prelude interventions. Most of these AMI prelude interventions consisted of only one or two sessions. Many of the studies they reviewed found significant effects for the AMI prelude on attendance in subsequent therapy and on drinking measures and measures of drug abuse. Burke (2002) reported an effect size of 0.21 for AMIs as stand-alone treatments and a considerably higher effect size of 0.53 for AMIs as a prelude to other treatments.

In a well-designed study that appeared after the meta-analysis, Connors, Walitzer, Dermen, et al. (2002) compared one 90-minute AMI prelude session to a 90-minute role induction prelude (to educate clients about what is expected of them and what they can expect in therapy) and to no prelude. Following this, all subjects received 12 individual and 12 group therapy sessions. These therapies were multicomponent interventions consisting of problem-solving and relapse prevention strategies, Alcoholics Anonymous, and other components, but did not include any further MI. The therapists who conducted the preludes were different from those who conducted the subsequent therapy sessions. The results provided strong support for the AMI prelude. Clients in the AMI prelude session attended more subsequent therapy sessions and had fewer heavy drinking days than did subjects who received no prelude, with the latter no different on these outcomes from those who received the role induction prelude session. The results of further analyses suggested that the AMI prelude exerted its effects partially, but not entirely, through its effect on session attendance. There has been only one report of the use of AMI as a prelude for problems other than alcohol and drug addiction. Treasure et al. (1999) compared four sessions of

CBT with four sessions of an AMI called motivational enhancement therapy (MET) and found that they were equally effective.

A recent study by Westra and Dozois (2004) represents the first randomized clinical trial of "pure" MI (i.e., without the feedback component) and with clinical disorders other than alcohol and substance abuse. Subjects for this study met diagnostic criteria for at least one anxiety disorder (either generalized anxiety disorder, panic disorder with or without agoraphobia, or social phobia). They were randomly assigned to receive either a three-session MI pretreatment (MIPT) or no pretreatment (NPT). Subsequently all subjects participated in group CBT for anxiety management. The MIPT group showed significantly greater reductions in their primary outcome measure of anxiety compared with the NPT group. In addition, the MIPT group scored significantly higher on a self-rating measure of homework compliance, although there were no differences on a therapist rating measure. MIPT subjects also significantly increased their scores on a measure of optimism for change from before to after the three sessions of MIPT. While 84% of the MIPT groups completed treatment compared to 63% of the NPT group, this difference only approached significance.

In summary, there is a considerable body of research to suggest that MI (or AMI in most cases) is reasonably effective for problems of alcohol and drug abuse as well as diet and exercise, with no significant effects found for smoking or HIV-risk behaviors. The strong results for AMIs as a prelude to other treatments suggest that this is a particularly promising area. The Westra and Dozois (2004) study provides support for the use of "pure" MI as a prelude to CBT for disorders other than those relating to alcohol and substance abuse.

If indeed a few sessions of MI preceding the main treatment significantly enhance the effect of that treatment by reducing ambivalence and increasing motivation, then we may have a powerful and widely applicable strategy. The application of ambivalence work as a prelude to the treatment of common clinical disorders other than the addictions is a very promising area for further research and clinical intervention.

SUMMARY

We have looked at length for therapy approaches that could be useful in the resolution of client ambivalence, and discuss those that we found.

While promising, they have a number of limitations as well. Most have little or no research support regarding their effectiveness, and some are hard to adapt into a therapist's existing approach. We believe that two approaches, the two-chair approach and MI, are especially suited to the resolution of ambivalence. They both foster a style and spirit that welcomes the client as a respected partner in the process of change. MI and the two-chair approach both have a body of trainable skills to assist therapists who are working with client ambivalence. Both have sufficient research support to suggest that they are effective models. These two therapies are clearly the most "on target" and we recommend that they be the interventions of choice when clients are struggling to resolve ambivalence.

CHAPTER 6

The Two-Chair Approach
Part I

The client, a woman in her early 40s with two young sons, had recently experienced an unexpected divorce. It had left her shaken and she was working hard to make sense out of what had happened and to cope with all the new challenges in her life. Her ex-husband had been caught in an affair. When she confronted him about the affair, he told her that he was divorcing her. After announcing his intention to divorce her, he became verbally abusive, extremely angry, and uncooperative with any of her efforts to understand what had gone wrong. Her attempts to interact with him left her feeling raw, abused, and lacking in self-esteem. She told the therapist that she knew she had to minimize contact with him and to disengage from him except for providing basic information about their children. Yet she continued to maintain contact with him, thereby suffering more verbal abuse and feelings of devastation.

In this example, we see the necessary conditions for the marker of ambivalence:

- She states that there is a behavior change on her part that would clearly be in her best interest—that is, to stop creating situations in which she ends up feeling abused.
- She believes that she has both the knowledge and the ability to make the change (e.g., stop making unnecessary phone calls to him, refuse to engage with him if he initiates the contact and becomes abusive).

TABLE 6.1. Steps in Working with the Two-Chair Approach

1. Identify the marker of ambivalence.
   a. Identify the specific ambivalence to be addressed.
   b. Present observations about the presence of ambivalence.
   c. Confirm the experience of the ambivalence with the client.
   d. Validate or normalize the client's experience when necessary.

2. Prepare to establish the two-chair experiment.
   a. Introduce the two-chair experiment with an appropriate rationale.
   b. Obtain a commitment of willingness from the client to enter the experiment.
   c. Assume a more directive role as therapist.
   d. Physically structure the experiment.
   e. Begin the actual experiment.

3. Foster and maintain a therapeutic dialogue in the present moment.
   a. Establish and maintain a clear experience of each discrepant self (separation).
   b. Establish and maintain a dialogue between the selves (contact).
   c. Encourage client's emotional arousal in both selves.

4. Resolution.
   a. Clarify the discrepancies and meanings of the ambivalence.
   b. Acknowledge and/or integrate discrepant self-schemas

Note. Adapted from Greenberg, Rice, and Elliott (1993). Copyright 1993 by The Guilford Press. Adapted by permission.

- But she is unable to get herself to make the changes even after renewed commitments to do so during therapy sessions.
- She feels badly about herself for not disengaging from him.

When there is a marker of ambivalence during a therapy session, a two-chair approach can be a useful intervention. Table 6.1 outlines the steps in using the two-chair approach with a marker of ambivalence.[1] This chapter and the next, where we discuss the steps of the two-chair approach, are not meant to be a full-fledged manual on the two-chair process. Our goal is to provide sufficient information to enable experi-

[1]We are indebted to the work of Leslie Greenberg and his associates for their development of the concept of "in-session markers" and their design of specific interventions for each marker. Our efforts are based solidly on their work (see Greenberg, Rice, & Elliott, 1993; Greenberg & Safran, 1987).

enced therapists to effectively use the two-chair approach when they deem it appropriate. We also hope that more novice therapists will find the approach valuable enough that they will pursue additional materials and training.

STEP 1: IDENTIFICATION OF THE MARKER OF AMBIVALENCE

Noting the Ambivalence

When the therapist observes a marker of ambivalence, he or she may share the observation with the client by saying something like "You seem to be very eager to stop destructive encounters with your ex-husband, yet you clearly haven't been able to find a way to do it" or "It seems that you move back and forth between the part of you that loves the challenge and pace of the corporate world, and a part of you that seeks a quieter, more spiritual life. And you haven't been able to feel totally comfortable in either place. It leaves you feeling distressed."

The therapist continually works toward achieving clarification and understanding of the client's world. The therapist also begins to direct attention to the client's current feelings, perceptions, and body sensations. This focus will teach the client how to attend to present-moment experience and prepare the client for the two-chair experiment.

Use the client's own language to speak about the ambivalence. If the client says, "Every time I try to help myself out of this situation I feel sad and lost and do nothing," the therapist might say something like "I hear you speak from a self that wants to get out of this relationship, and a self that feels sad, lost, and afraid to leave. It's as if there are two of you, one wanting to be free and one afraid to move." Using the client's own language facilitates the client's experience of being understood and also promotes the client's full experience of his or her thoughts and feelings.

Confirming the Experience of Ambivalence with the Client

The therapist needs to confirm the accuracy of the observation that ambivalence is present. For example, the therapist might ask, "So, there is a part of you that believes it's important to follow your doctor's recommendations, and a part of you that doesn't seem to be able to do it. Am I hearing you correctly?" Or the therapist might remark, "A part of you seems to know that you would be happier and less depressed if you spend more time with others, and yet you just can't seem to bring yourself to do that. Is this your experience?" It is important that both the therapist and the client have a clear and correct understanding of the ambivalence. The client is the "expert" as to whether or not the therapist's observations fit. If the client does not agree with the therapist's observations, the two of them need to work together to clarify the issue and arrive at a mutual understanding. They become partners in defining and refining the client's experience (as it changes within a session or over time), necessitating a continuing collaboration to understand the client's present experience.

Validating or Normalizing the Client's Experience

The therapist communicates that it is normal for people to experience ambivalence, and notes that such ambivalence tells us that we are being pulled in different directions that we need to understand. Occasionally a client expresses concern when we introduce the idea of voices or selves. If needed, we assure him or her that when we refer to disparate "selves" we are not talking about dissociative identity disorder, or multiple personality disorder. Our use of the term "separate selves" reflects the multivoiced experience described by Bromberg (1998), Hermans (1996), Honos-Webb and Stiles (1998), and others. It is a common experience that we all have when we are of more than one mind about something.

For example, a client reported that he had a very difficult time expanding his world beyond an endless routine of going to work and going home. For several years he had wanted to explore the surrounding sights, but he spent every weekend stuck in place. He knew that his world was very narrow and that it would be good for him to involve himself in different activities and to risk more involvement with other people. He felt sad that he wanted to do many things but couldn't bring himself to do any of them. He felt in a persistent state of struggle with himself.

Regarding the case example described at the beginning of this chapter, the therapist might say: "I know it must be terribly hard for you. You never expected to be abandoned by your husband, and although interactions with him are very hurtful, I see a part of you that wants to rescue the relationship and a part of you that wants to stop being abused. This is a dilemma that many people would feel in your situation."

STEP 2: PREPARATION FOR THE EXPERIMENT

Introducing the Experiment with an Appropriate Rationale

Once the therapist and the client agree that ambivalence is present and has been accurately understood, the therapist introduces the experiment. The therapist might say something like "Would you be willing to try an exercise right now that may help us to better understand your mixed feelings and perhaps help facilitate change?" If the client responds with a clear "Yes," the therapist proceeds with the experiment. But if the client reveals any hesitation or asks to know more about the nature of the experiment, further discussion and clarification is necessary.

It is important to provide the client with a rationale for the experiment. Without it, clients are understandably reluctant to do anything that is different from what they expect in therapy. Clients generally expect to "talk about" things with the therapist, so the invitation to enter into an in-session experiment may make them uneasy. A *rationale* is a clear and succinct statement about why you are asking the client to do the exercise. For example, you might say:

> "I find that it often helps to better understand what is going on if we find a way to clearly express both sides of the issue you've been experiencing. There is the part of you that seems to be saying that you want very much to date and the part of you that shrinks from opportunities to date. It is often useful to separate those two parts of yourself by using two chairs and creating a dialogue between the parts. This may help us both to better understand the two sides of your ambivalence. Would you be willing to try this?"

Sometimes clients are hesitant, based on their own internal predictions about what will happen if they enter the experiment. These predictions may include "I'll feel totally embarrassed," "I'm afraid that I'll make a fool of myself," "I won't know what to say," or "This feels strange." The therapist should acknowledge and normalize those experiences: "Yes, sometimes it feels a little awkward at first; however, I find that people almost always get beyond that. Remember, also, that you are in charge and you can stop the experiment at any time."

We find that with such reassurances, clients usually agree to try the experiment. However, we have occasionally seen students of this technique exaggerate the "strangeness" of the experiment and actually talk clients out of doing it. I (DEE) supervised clinical students and from time to time suggested appropriate in-session experiments, such as the two-chair dialogue, to use with their clients. Sometimes the response was "I don't think my client is ready for that." When I probed a bit, I often found that the "unreadiness" was a projection on the part of the student. Once these students were convinced of the possible usefulness of the experiment and became comfortable with it, they were able to discuss the experiment with their clients in such a way that most agreed to try it.

Using Alternatives When Appropriate

We acknowledge that there are some clients who are not willing to try the experiment, or who are willing to try but do not profit from it. In such cases, we recommend that the therapist discontinue efforts to engage the client in the two-chair experiment and consider alternate approaches, such as those discussed in Chapter 5. Another possibility is to use a slightly different technique that we have found to be helpful when the client is uncomfortable with the two-chair experiment, which is playing "devil's advocate." When a therapist is clear about the client's reluctance to do the two-chair experiment, the therapist may play one of the selves (either the Change Self or the No-Change Self), with the client playing the other. The dialogue is between two live people rather than between the client and a "self" in an empty chair. First the therapist identifies and confirms the presence of separate selves—as is always done in the two-chair approach. Then the therapist offers to play one of the selves. If the client agrees, the therapist moves to one of the chairs designated for the two-chair experiment.

Choosing which self to play is based on the therapist's sense of which self the client is having most difficulty articulating (e.g., in terms of thoughts, feelings, wants, or needs). In psychodrama, if another person steps into such a role, the client sometimes gives specific instructions about what to say and how to say it. Here, the therapist tries to adopt the worldview of the client's portrayed self and to engage in a dialogue with the client as if taking part in a spontaneous two-person conversation.

The therapist's tone depends upon his or her knowledge of the client. With one client who grew up on the streets of Philadelphia, it was very helpful to be confronting and challenging to the self in the other chair. He was able to respond in kind and felt comfortable with this kind of strong give-and-take. Seldom did he concede a point or change a position while engaged in the experiment, but sometimes he showed a shift in his position in subsequent sessions.

While engaging in the devil's advocate interaction, the therapist has a dual role as a participant in the interaction and as a therapist. The therapist often has to step outside of the experiment to check with the client about the usefulness of the experiment and about any cognitive or emotional shifts that are occurring. In a group or in the presence of another therapist, the therapist can enlist either another group member or the other therapist to play the role of the devil's advocate. In either case, it is important to clearly establish where the experiment begins and ends and to reestablish the person who played the role as an individual separate from the role that was being played. Using chairs designated specifically for the two-chair dialogue keeps roles separate—the physical movement into and out of the experiment chairs identifies a shift in role.

Discussing Concerns

It may be valuable, when clients are hesitant, to scale down the intervention before inviting the client into the two-chair experiment. For example, a warm-up exercise consists of having the client first speak from each "side" of the ambivalence without moving from his or her original chair. After the warm-up, the client may be less reluctant to use the two chairs. If, on the other hand, the client still does not want to enter into the two-chair experiment, the therapist must respect that decision and move on to other interventions.

Once a client has agreed to enter into the experiment, it is helpful for him or her to label or describe the two parts of the divided self. Clients who are ambivalent may not conceptualize the issue in terms of a divided self with distinct and different positions, so this "naming" will help them to do so. The naming often leads to a sense of relief because they can now make more sense of the fact that they've been unable to make a desired change. Most people need some instruction and support to learn how to identify and name the selves. Sometimes clients will spontaneously name the two voices. Many will simply label the discrepant selves as "Wants to Change" and "Opposes Change," or "Positive" and "Negative." For example, one client referred to one side as "Healthy" and the other side as "Stubborn." In the case discussed at the beginning of this chapter, the therapist suggested labels of "Seeks Disengagement" and "Stays Engaged." The client confirmed that these labels "felt right." Later they had to redefine the selves as they evolved. In another case, the authors worked with a man who found it useful to describe the two parts of himself by the last name of his father's family and the last name of his mother's family, respectively. The mother's family tended toward obesity, and he felt that the part of him that would not cooperate in losing weight was more aligned with that side. The part of him that wanted to lose weight was more aligned with his father's family. These labels proved very useful in working with his ambivalence about losing weight.

Accurate identification of the different selves is very important in this process. Let us return to the opening case, where the client was stunned by her husband's affair and sudden decision to divorce her. She participated for two or three sessions in a two-chair dialogue between a Seeks Disengagement Self and Stays Engaged Self. Her identified goal was to stop allowing her husband to verbally abuse her. Although she left each session resolved to disengage, she failed to do so and the two-chair work did not appear to be helping.

Subsequently, the therapist returned to empathic client-centered exploration. In the process, the client recalled a time when she was a child living with her single-parent mother. Her father, from a working-class New England family, had abruptly left the family. She described a scene in which she felt very emotional and desperate. Her mother had scolded her and her sister and had sent them to their rooms. In the most vivid part of this memory, she wrote little notes saying that she was sorry and slipped them under the door. She fervently sought forgiveness and reconnection with her mother. She was asked if she could make any connection between these experiences and the current situation with her husband. She could, and then spoke about how careful and resolved she had been to choose a husband who would never leave her as her father had left the family. She had dated several different men, each for long periods of time, trying to discern if each man could remain absolutely faithful to their relationship. Only when she felt totally confident did she decide to marry the man she did. Now that he was divorcing her, her trust in herself had been devastated. A divorce would mean that one of her most carefully crafted decisions was absolutely wrong. She wondered how she could ever be certain of anything again.

Once this pivotal experience was in the open, we returned to the ambivalence, but with some redefinitions. Now the two selves were identified as the self that seeks disengagement from her husband's abuse (Disengage Self) and the self that fights frantically to preserve her sense of competency, needing to stay married as a way to preserve her sense of sound judgment (Frantic Self). In the dialogue that followed, the Disengage Self began to remind her of other parts of her life in which she was and is competent—as a parent and as a professional, as well as someone who was an expert on antique porcelains. Slowly she began to accept her competence, and began to acknowledge that a failure in one area was not a failure in all areas. Over the next few sessions, she began to disengage from her husband. At one point, she brought her two sons to a session so that the therapist could see that they were bright, happy, and well-adjusted children. This helped to strengthen her experience of a competent self that could better disengage from the relationship with her husband. It was only when we correctly understood and labeled the different selves that the experiment led to actual change in her life.

The Therapist's Role during the Experiment

Once the two-chair experiment is introduced, the therapist must shift toward a *more active and directive position*, without neglecting to maintain an empathic stance. The therapist must do enough "coaching" and directing to help structure the experiment and to keep it moving along, without "leading" the client to specific experiences or conclusions. The therapist's role is to facilitate the emergence and expression of those thoughts, tendencies, and feelings that occur during the course of the experiment. The therapist's task is to continually seek information from the client by carefully monitoring his or her verbal and nonverbal cues. Emerging or stifled emotions are particularly important to monitor.

In this part of the work, the therapist's interventions are largely confined to directives and observations. The therapist generally avoids asking questions during the experiment because questions call for a response on the part of the client, which may interrupt the therapy process. If the client turns away from the dialogue with the empty chair, the therapist must move the client back into the experiment.

Of course, there will be times during the experiment when the therapist needs to gather information. Rather than interrupting the process with a question, the therapist can obtain the same information by turning the question into a directive. For example, instead of asking "What are you feeling now?", the therapist could say, "Tell the other part of yourself how you are feeling as you say that." Table 6.2 presents some examples of shared observations and directives.

In the following dialogue, the therapist and the client have determined that there is both a Shy Self and an Outgoing Self. The therapist shares observations and gives directives that keep the client focused on her moment-to-moment experience and foster the engagement of both

TABLE 6.2. Types of Therapist Observations and Directives with Examples

Therapist observations and directives	Examples
Therapist observations	
1. About behavior	"I notice that you began to report some resentment and then you changed the subject."
	"I am aware that you were not able to follow the plan we set up, and I am curious to understand the part of you that has difficulty with the plan."
2. About body reactions	"When you sit here, you look as if you want to get very small and shrink into the chair."
	"You look scared, as if you want to run out of the room."
3. About voice tone	"Notice that you speak to the other part of you like a parent scolding a child."
	"You sound discouraged and ready to give up as you talk to her."
Therapist directives	
1. Directed toward managing the experiment itself	"Good, now come and sit in this chair and respond to what that part just said."
	"You are talking to me, and I'd like to have you say that again, but say it to the part of you in the other chair."
2. Directed toward helping the client experiment with a new behavior, position, or attitude	"Say more about this part of you—the part that gets scared to make a move."
	"You sound very frustrated. See if you can get a full sense of that frustration, and say more about it."

Note. Adapted from Greenberg, Rice, and Elliott (1993). Copyright 1993 by The Guilford Press. Adapted by permission.

parts of her self in dialogue. The transcript picks up at the point where the client has agreed to the two-chair experiment, has moved into one of the chairs, and is waiting for direction.

THERAPIST: Okay. I'm going to invite you to have a conversation between those two sides of yourself, and just let me listen in to that conversation as you talk. Just speak the dialogue . . . the dialogue that you do back and forth in your head all the time. [Giving instruction and some rationale]

CLIENT: Uh-huh.

THERAPIST: I'm just inviting you to do it in the open. That way it helps you to slow it [the internal dialogue] down enough to pay attention to what really goes on in that dialogue. And it also gives you a chance to get clear about the different parts of yourself, okay? [Expanding rationale]

CLIENT: Okay. (*Sits in the chair designated as the Outgoing Self.*)

THERAPIST: What do you want to say to this shy part of yourself sitting over here? [Gesturing to the empty chair, and giving a directive]

OUTGOING SELF: Well, there is really no reason for you to be so shy. A little bit of shyness is fine, but you can't have fun if you just pull back and keep within yourself. You are shy to the extreme. People don't want to be around you if you're going to be quiet all the time.

THERAPIST: Come over here and be this part of you. [Giving a directive]

SHY SELF: Okay. Well, I may not be as much fun as you want me to be . . . but then I don't get negative responses back in case they don't like me, and it just keeps me out of trouble. [Change in facial expression and voice tone imply that this side has some fearfulness]

THERAPIST: There seem to be some feelings connected to why you're shy. Will you tell her about that? [Sharing an observation and giving a directive]

The Experiment Follows the Client's Lead

In the directive stance illustrated above, the therapist doesn't know exactly where the client should go and doesn't lead the client toward a particular goal or outcome. The therapist only facilitates those actions and behaviors that keep the client focused on and engaged in the two-chair dialogue. The position taken here is that an experiment is truly that: an experiment. The outcome is unknown, so both client and therapist must approach it with the open attitude of learning from it. All emerging information is potentially useful.

The discovery function of the two-chair experiment does not involve attending to *why* emotions, behaviors, or cognitions came to be, but to an *awareness* that they are present. The experiment creates the conditions under which the client generates his or her own meaning. The therapist helps the client access moment-to-moment experience in a manner that allows for a clear understanding of the conflicting self-schemas and the emergence of new personal meanings. Therapists who take an inquisitive, curious, "not knowing" position are more likely to avoid the temptation to create their own meaning for the client.

The Experiment as a Continued Assessment

There is a client assessment before the experiment begins and the experiment itself continues to be an assessment. For example, neither the client nor the therapist may understand the very demanding quality of one self or the fearfulness of another self until these selves are observed in interaction in the two-chair dialogue.

At times, the new information provided by the experiment can be dramatic. The authors once worked with a young woman who had recently experienced the breakup of a romantic relationship. When we asked her about how she was doing with that loss, she indicated that she was "doing fine." We suggested an empty-chair experiment and asked her to place the ex-boyfriend in an empty chair for a moment. Her immediate response was crying. Then her emotions changed to resentment toward him. Subsequently in that session she reported feeling relieved, and in the next session she stated that she felt more resolved about the situation. Without the experiment, we might have moved on, believing that she was doing well after the breakup of her relationship.

Physically Structuring the Experiment

Once the therapist has a clear commitment from the client to enter into the experiment, the therapist physically arranges the room so that two empty chairs are opposite one another. It is a good idea to use two chairs that are alike so that any physical differences that the client experiences in moving from one chair to the other will be due to a psychological shift in his or her experience rather than to the physical characteristics of the chairs (e.g., soft vs. hard). If possible, it is also a good idea to use two different chairs from the ones in which the therapist and the client sit while engaged in conversation with each other. The client's movement from the original chair into the two additional chairs marks the beginning of the experiment. The client's movement back to his or her original seat indicates a clear end to the experiment for that session.

Valuing the Moment-to-Moment Client Experience

The client often develops an early explanation for his or her difficulty in changing. We try to redirect the client away from premature conclusions as to "why" something is happening and toward "what" is happening until the underlying cognitive and emotional structures are brought to light and clarified. If the client focuses on present experience, he or she will eventually be able to provide his or her own meaning for these experiences, one that is grounded more solidly in what unfolds in the experiment.

We are not minimizing the role of cognitive understanding. It is crucial that clients develop new understanding or create new meanings in this work. Clients often make spontaneous connections that create solid insight. One client, at the end of a dialogue between an extremely critical Should Self and a battered, criticized Fearful Self, while sitting in the Should Self chair, said, "I just realized that when I sit here, I am my mother!" This spontaneous insight changed her understanding of what was going on and motivated her toward better self-support and change. If no new understanding or awareness emerges, the therapist may prompt it with such questions as "What meaning do you give to what you just experienced in the experiment?" or "What is different about your understanding now?"

Observing the Contrasts

Therapist observations of the client's process can provide valuable information. For example, the therapist may recognize that the client's voice in one chair is clear and assertive, while the client's voice in the other chair sounds subdued and powerless. Or the therapist may notice that the client sounds like a scolding parent in one chair, while he or she appears younger and sulking in the other. These observations can lead to productive interventions. The therapist needs to be especially attentive to nonverbal behaviors and to discrepancies between verbal and nonverbal expressions.

The therapist can look for shifts in the client's experience that are indicative of therapeutic change (e.g., a softening of voice tone, a hint of a rising emotion that is quickly terminated, or a sigh of relief). When these shifts do occur, the therapist encourages them by directing the client to stay with them until they are fully experienced.

Facilitating the Expression of One Emotion at a Time

As the client engages in the two-chair experiment he or she may experience, various feelings that surface and seek expression. As long as they are clearly experienced and expressed, the experiment continues apace. However, if the client is trying to express more than one primary emotion at a time, there is a real possibility of client confusion and feelings of being stuck. Just as we assist a person in identifying separate selves, we also assist him or her in learning to separate different emotions and to give each emotion its own expression. When a mixture of emotional states arises, it will often be apparent to the therapist that one of the emotions has a stronger attachment to one of the selves than to the other.

For example, a client might verbally express resentment, while his or her nonverbal cues suggest sadness and tears. Here, we have the presence of both resentment and sadness. The therapist can bring this to the client's attention with a comment like "See if you feel resentful or sad right now. Let yourself experience the one that seems stronger and speak from that feeling. If or when the other feeling emerges as stronger, go with it."

A person may have to practice expressing emotions so that both the verbal and the nonverbal expressions are in harmony. Some people will remark that they have some awareness that they use tears to express everything, as if all emotions go to a "default setting" of sadness or anger or shame. They may typically be unaware of their emotional "one note" expression so that they do not know what to make of it or how to change it. For example, one of us (DEE) worked with a woman who identified an ambivalence marker, agreed to the two-chair experiment, and was ready to begin. Before going any further she asked for a tissue and told the therapist that she knew that she was going to cry—this in face of the fact that she had been speaking more about resentment than sadness. Throughout the experiment the therapist carefully tracked each time when she began to cry and intervened by requesting each time that she tell the other self if she currently felt more hurt or more angry. Soon, she was able to report "I caught myself about to cry again, but I'm really still angry." Then she was able to express her resentments with appropriate voice tone and posture.

Chapter 7 addresses the next two steps of the two-chair approach. Step 3 discusses the actual heart of the dialogue and the two essential components of good dialogue: separation and contact. Step 4 discusses how resolution occurs.

SUMMARY

In this chapter we have discussed how to identify a marker of ambivalence and share it with clients. We also discussed the importance of confirming the validity of observations about ambivalence with the client and normalizing the experience of ambivalence. Then we described how to introduce the two-chair approach and the importance of obtaining consent to engage in the experiment. The chapter also addressed the shifting role of the therapist in the experiment, from relatively non-directive to a more directive and facilitating role.

The chapter included helpful suggestions derived from our clinical experience as practitioners of the approach and as instructors to students. These had to do with the importance of correctly naming the different selves, the need to have an understandable rationale for introducing the experiment, and the value of exploring client predictions about entering an experiment. We also described the use of observations and directives as important methods to bring the experiment to life. We dwelt on the importance of following the client lead and of allowing the client to arrive at a new emotional meaning. Finally, we suggested playing the "devil's advocate" as an alternative strategy for those times when it is appropriate.

CHAPTER 7

The Two-Chair Approach

Part II

STEP 3: THE TWO-CHAIR DIALOGUE

Establishing and Maintaining Separate Voices

The internal dialogue that people experience can sometimes be like the rumblings of a mob—many voices pressing for attention all at once, making each separate voice indistinguishable. Consider the example of two warring nations attempting to meet at the peace table. If members of each delegation yelled whatever and whenever they felt like it, the result would be cacophony—a loud noise of discordant and indeterminate voices. In two-chair work, the sides need to be separated so that the nature of the opposing sides becomes clear. In the early stages of this work, the goal of the therapist is to help the client identify the conflicting sides and separate them so that all of the forces pulling one way are consolidated in one chair, while all the forces pulling the other way are seated in the other chair. Once the selves have been identified and separated, the focus shifts to contact and engagement. Both selves begin to appreciate the nature of the wants and needs of the other side, evoking a true dialogue.

At times, we find that a dominant and vocal part of the self demands change, and the self that opposes change doesn't have much of a voice. In these situations, the therapist has to create conditions where the fledgling side can find its wings.

A 40-year-old divorced woman had an on-again, off-again relationship with her ex-husband. They lived together for short periods of time,
and then one of them would find reason to leave. When the concept of
ambivalence was introduced, she identified with it immediately, saying
that it was exactly what she did in her head—that she talks back and
forth and even on occasion writes from the two different positions, to
either stay in or to leave the relationship.

Helping Clients Establish the Voices

In their internal dialogue, people may cycle from one self to the other so
rapidly that they are unaware of the shifts. In the two-chair dialogue, it is
common for a client to begin a sentence by speaking from one self and
to finish it with content that belongs to the other self. The therapist
monitors these switches from one self to the other and prompts the client to change chairs when the switches happen. For example:

SAD SELF: (*expressing sadness about always being pushed by the side that wants
to change*) I'm sad that you can't understand when I need a break.
I'm only able to do so much, and sometimes I feel exhausted. I
know that if I didn't keep pushing there is a chance that nothing
would get done.

THERAPIST: I think you just switched to the other part of yourself.
Come into the other chair and say the last sentence again.

DESIRED SELF: (*from the other chair*) Yes, if I didn't push you nothing
would get done.

THERAPIST: (*teaching the client how to monitor the changes from one self-
schema to another*) Just keep in mind that there appears to be a part
of you that pushes and a part of your that is tired and sad. Notice
that you quickly switch from one part to the other. Tell her again
why you push so hard, and then move to the other chair and respond.

Clients are often amazed at how they experience the different
selves in the two chairs. They become aware of physical differences in
the experience of each chair: they may speak in a different tone, sit with
a different posture, feel stronger in one chair and weaker in the other,
and so on. Sometimes they find themselves comfortable and "safe" in
one chair and reluctant to sit in the other. Some clients express alarm

about the existence of such contrasting selves, believing that it may be a sign of "craziness." Gentle reassurance on the part of the therapist can easily put such fears to rest.

Signs of Good Separation

There are several indicators that the client has achieved separation between the different selves.

Separate Content. One is that the content in one chair is clearly differentiated from the content in the other. The following example is from an early session with a man very recently confined to a wheelchair. He vacillated between an overly optimistic self that believed, contrary to medical evidence, that he would be able to walk again and do all the things that able-bodied people do, and a depressed self who believed that he would never walk again.

DESIRED SELF: (*excitement in his voice*) I know that with a little more effort you can do that again. You just need to work out more and exercise your legs more. . . . When you do that, people won't see you as disabled . . . you'll have an easier time getting into a relationship. Your life will really take off.

THERAPIST: See how the other part of you responds to that.

DEPRESSED SELF: (*subdued voice*) You're kidding yourself . . . I know it isn't going to happen. I feel like giving up. I've been depressed for weeks now, and your attempts to promise me my life back won't work. Face it . . . I keep thinking how much better off I'd be if I were dead.

The therapist checked after the experiment ended for any suicidal ideation.

Self-Recognition. A second indicator of good separation occurs when clients recognize, in the middle of a sentence, that the other part of the self is beginning to speak. Clients will either tell the therapist that the other part of the self is beginning to speak or they will spontaneously move to the other chair to speak from the part of the self that has come into focus. The next example involves a client who was ambivalent about keeping her new job:

SHOULD SELF: I believe you can succeed at your new job. It takes time to learn any new job, and you've only been there 3 weeks. Remember that it took you months to know everything about your previous job. Relax and give yourself some time. (*Pauses and then speaks to the therapist.*) I'm beginning to hear the negative part of me again and I need to move over there. (*Points to and moves to the other chair.*)

DISCOURAGED SELF: I just don't think I can do it. I've had to stay late . . . very late every day to get my work done. No one else has to stay late. I'm totally exhausted at the end of a day . . . and too tired to attend to things in my apartment (defeated voice). I think I made a bad choice in taking this job. (*Silently gets up and moves back to the other chair.*)

SHOULD SELF: I think you forget that you felt the same way on your last job . . . remember that it took you a while to get the hang of it. You have a long weekend coming up and you can use that time to regroup. Give it a few months and see how it goes.

Nonverbal Confirmation. In the above example, nonverbal behaviors were also different in each chair. This client experienced the two selves as relatively clear and distinct. She looked firm and supportive (although a little frustrated) when she spoke from the Should Self. In contrast, she appeared and sounded very sad and depressed when speaking from the Discouraged Self.

Equality of Selves or Voices

Frequently, in the early stages of two-chair work, one side is expressed clearly and strongly, while the other side is weak and vague. The self that seeks change usually understands the need for change and has a clear position. The self that resists change is often less well understood and articulated. The therapist listens for signs of emergence of the weaker/confused part and supports that side until it expresses itself more clearly and forcefully. For example, the therapist may say: "She seems to have a good grasp on the reasons you should be doing something about your health situation. But I'm less clear about the part of you that finds that difficult to do. . . . Please come and sit over here and tell her what you can about the difficulty."

Establishing and Maintaining Good Contact

The next step is to foster contact between the selves. *Contact* is the engagement of one part of the self with the other. The therapist looks for the same signs of engagement that one finds in a productive dialogue between two different people: facial expressions, body posture, voice tone, emotionality, and so on. Without the experience of contact, the client may go through the motions of doing an experiment without deriving any new insight from it.

Contact typically leads to greater emotional experience, which makes it easier to access schema-related material (Arkowitz & Hanna, 1989; Beck & Weishaar, 1989; Greenberg & Safran, 1987). Once elicited, it is available to the client for modification (Greenberg et al., 1993). Without good contact between the selves, there can be no resolution of the ambivalence.

Importance of Contact

Like good contact between two people, good contact between different selves includes respect, mutuality, and an appreciation of the beliefs and feelings of the other self. It also includes acceptance of what the other self expresses and a sense that the different selves are engaged in a common effort. Good contact between different voices reveals needs, values, and motivations that facilitate the emergence of new meanings, choices, and solutions.

Modes of Poor Contact

In describing modes of "poor contact" we are not implying that they can or ought to be avoided. They will occur. As they do, we bring them to the client's awareness so that he or she can experiment with more productive contact. Remember that all the data are useful and "friendly."

Parent–Child Interaction (or a Should Self and a Reactant Self). One self assumes a parenting role and the other self takes on the response mode of the child. When the "parenting self" is loving, nurturing, and listening, there is less struggle between the selves. By contrast, when the Parenting Self takes on a blaming or scolding tone, the dialogue can become circular or nonproductive. These attitudes evoke a number of different child-like responses. The Child Self may feel defeated and give up, believing that any assertion of needs is fruitless. The Child Self can whine and complain, without ever stating what it needs in order to feel cared for. Or the Child Self may get stuck in a generalized, poorly understood, negative feeling state or state of confusion.

Sometimes the parent–child interaction is a replay of the client's actual interactions with his or her parents or other significant adults. People may do to themselves what others have done to them without even being aware that this is happening. Over the course of a two-chair experiment, they can become aware that this is happening. This awareness can be helpful in developing more accepting and nurturing behavior toward the self.

One of us (DEE) once worked with a client who revealed that she criticized almost everything she did. She agreed to the two-chair experiment involving the Criticizing Self in one chair and the Criticized Self in another. A dialogue ensued manifested little feeling or progress until the Criticized Self said to the Criticizing Self that she was "just like Dad." When the therapist suggested that she repeat her remark, she began to cry and to talk about what it was like to be subjected to her father's criticism. She had been unable to acknowledge the effect his criticism had on her because she believed that it was "motivated by love." She began to distinguish the effects her father's behavior had on her from his motivation, which allowed her to express long-withheld emotional reactions about her father. The therapist suggested an experiment during the following week in which she was to remind herself, when she was being self-critical, that she was "being just like Dad." Therapy subsequently focused on helping her become more self-nurturant and less self-critical.

Cognitive Debate. Another mode of poor contact takes the form of a *cognitive debate*, with an almost complete absence of affect. The tone is one of competitive one-upmanship, with each side trying to "score points" against the other. Both sides line up their reasons and make their points, but make little movement toward any kind of resolution. It looks as if they are engaged, because the selves are actively debating with one another, but they are not engaged. This situation is reminiscent of working with a couple in which the partners are trapped in a stale, mechanical exchange of old complaints, with both feeling certain that they're right. Each partner repeats his or her position, believing that in time the other person will "come around." Both in work with couples and in the two-chair approach, the task is to increase emotional experience and enliven the dialogue so that it is fresh and present-centered. The therapist can ask each self to make an emotional response to what the other self has just said. A particularly useful intervention is to give this directive: "Tell the other side how what he [or she] just said makes you feel."

Disconnected Monologues. In cognitive debate, there is at least some slight contact with and acknowledgment of the other side. However, sometimes there is a total lack of connection between the selves. During couple therapy, we have witnessed couples in which both parties continue to tell their story almost as if the other party was not even present. This can also happen in two-chair work when one self does not even acknowledge the presence or experience of the other. It is as if the different selves live in two worlds, isolated from one another. One self speaks, but not to the other. Each waits its turn, has its say, then retreats and turns a deaf ear to what the other self is saying.

In the following example, the client begins to realize that a demanding, criticizing part of the self is just like her father. She describes what it is like to be under that kind of attack. However, the other part of the self continues in her demanding posture, unaffected by any reports of negative results:

WEAK SELF: (*weak voice*) I know that you are just like dad.

THERAPIST: Tell her more about that. [Giving a directive]

WEAK SELF: You're like Dad when you rail at me and tell me I'm lazy. You're like Dad when you scream at me. You're like Dad when you beat me up just because you don't have anybody else to take your frustrations out on. You're like Dad because you don't offer me the support I need right now. I couldn't live up to his expectations, and I can't live up to yours.

THERAPIST: Tell her what happens to you when she does those things. [Giving a directive]

WEAK SELF: I just feel hopeless and defeated. There's no way I can succeed, so I quit. I just quit. (*Tears begin to form in her eyes and she looks very sad.*)

THERAPIST: (*in a supportive voice*) Tell her about the tears. [Giving a directive]

WEAK SELF: I'm just so sad that I can't ever do anything right in your eyes.

THERAPIST: (*managing the experiment, waits while she deeply experiences the sadness, and then says*) Change to the other chair.

SHOULD SELF: (*totally ignoring the experience of the Weak Self*) I'm not going to apologize for being like Dad (*defiant voice*) because he was strong and he got through some tough times . . . and I get us through some tough times. And I don't want to apologize for that. But this is a tough time for you too and you need to do this. (*somewhat angry*) You need to change the way you think about stuff. And you can do it. It has nothing to do with meeting my expectations . . . you can do it. I know that it's there. But I just don't understand why you don't try harder.

The Should Self is entrenched and convinced of her position. She does not yet understand that her unrelenting efforts have the effect of causing the other part of the self to feel hopeless and to quit. The therapist's task is to keep the dialogue going and to encourage each self to respond to what the other self is saying. In this example, the therapist tried to get the Should Self to respond to the Weak Self's feelings of helplessness and sadness, and the Weak Self to begin to acknowledge the Should Self's fear of becoming nonfunctional.

Intervening to Create Productive Dialogues

A basic intervention is for the therapist to offer, in a nonjudgmental and tentative manner, observations about the exchange between the two parts. This intervention helps bring the client toward greater awareness, creating the possibility of experimentation with new behaviors. Remember that the therapist views the client as the expert. The therapist's observations are presented tentatively, subject to the client's approval and endorsement.

> "I get a sense, as I listen to the two parts of you talk, that it is somewhat like what I hear between parents and children. Continue the dialogue for a moment or two more and see if that rings true for you."

Interventions based on accurate observations enliven the dialogue. For example, the therapist may suggest that the client play each part to the hilt. For example, he or she may ask the scolding Parenting Self to experiment by shaking a finger at the Child Self and speaking in an even harsher voice. Then he or she might ask the client to switch and be the scolded Child Self and to portray the effect of being scolded. Such exaggerations of gestures and voice tone in each role can enable the client to experiment with changing the style or tone of the dialogue.

Fostering Emotional Arousal

Emotional arousal is an important aspect of our two-chair approach. We believe that emotional arousal facilitates bringing schematic material to awareness. Once in awareness, the schematic structures are more amenable to modification (Daldrup, Engle, Holiman, & Beutler, 1994).

When the two discrepant selves begin to experience and express their emotions, the quality of the contact seems to change dramatically. It is as if the music has been added to the lyrics. There are dramatic shifts in voice tone, statements are more thoughtful and nuanced, and the dialogue becomes deeper and more productive. Sometimes the increase in emotional arousal will be fleeting, necessitating quick intervention on the part of the therapist. If he or she notices a moistening of the eyes, a frustrated shuffle of feet, or a passing look of defeat, the therapist encourages the client to "stay with" that momentary experience until its presence is more clearly acknowledged and experienced. Or the therapist can say, "Tell him what just went on inside you when your eyes briefly moistened."

On rare occasions the emotional experience is very painful for the client. We must always work to stay within the comfort level of the client. It the person begins to express emotions in a way that appears to be very distressing, the therapist needs to clarify the situation. That can be done by inquiring whether the discomfort is acceptable to the client or whether the client is becoming overwhelmed and wants to stop.

Process-experiential therapists have gathered together a number of interventions that can be used to introduce and heighten emotional expression within the two-chair dialogue (Greenberg et al., 1993). Our clinical work has pointed us in the direction of other interventions that also assist in the development and expression of emotional content. We present a list of these interventions in Table 7.1 and briefly describe each type of intervention in this sections that follow.

TABLE 7.1. Interventions to intensify emotional experience.

Therapist intervention	Examples
1. Directing a person's attention	"Attend to what is going on in your body as you say that." "Notice that you hold your breath when you speak about your fear."
2. Sharing observations of the client	"I notice that you look small . . . that you seem to almost disappear as you try to respond to her." "You suddenly look sad . . . stay with that feeling and give it words when you can."
3. Developing language of ownership	"I'm aware that you qualify many of the things you say with words like *sort of* and *maybe*. Experiment with dropping the qualifying words and see what happens." "Change the word *it* to *I* and say that statement again."
4. Developing specifics and details	"Let yourself say more about the sadness. Tell him [the other self in the other chair] all the things that you are sad about." "You just said that you were 'fed up.' Tell him exactly what makes you 'fed up.'"
5. Exaggerating	"That sounds very important. Say it again and see if you can support it with a stronger voice. . . . Again, even stronger this time." "See if you can say that again in a less timid way."
6. Repeating	"Say that again. Repeat it several times and just allow yourself to experience what it is like to feel so misunderstood." "That sounded like a critical revelation. Say it again and hear what you are saying."
7. Changing position	"Try standing when you speak as the Strong Self and sitting when you speak from the Weak Self." "You're slumped each time you sit in this chair. Experiment with a different posture and see what happens."
8. Exploring restraint	"You begin to express your anger and then you squeeze it off. Notice what happens in your body as you do that. Pay attention to your muscles and your gut." "Continue to hold the feeling down and tell me what happens."
9. Exploring predictions	"You had a fleeting look on your face and then put it away. Tell the other part what you think would happen if you expressed that feeling." "From time to time you look angry for an instant. Tell me what you think will happen if you express that anger."
10. Eliciting emotional responses	"Tell him [the other self in the other chair] how you feel when he speaks to you that way." "How do you feel toward her when she is continually noncompliant with her meds?"
11. Suggesting "try-on" lines	"Say to the other part of yourself, 'I'm tired of you pushing me around all the time.'" "Say to that self: 'I depend on you and I am scared.'"

Directing a Person's Attention

Some clients follow their emotions naturally, reporting frequently on their emotional state, while others are either unaware or only partially aware of their feelings. To evoke emotional experiences, we direct the client to attend to those cues that may signal the presence of feeling states. In many cases, there are nonverbal cues. Such cues might involve noticing even small changes in the client's facial expressions, voice tone, posture, and so on, and asking that the client simply become aware of, or *attend* to, that change as it happens. For example, the therapist might remark "Be aware of your voice right now," or "Without changing it, notice your posture as you sit in this chair," or "Notice that each time you sit in this chair you hold your breath." When the therapist sees some change in the client that appears to be outside the client's awareness, the therapist simply asks the client to attend to that change.

Once the client is in the two-chair experiment, *suggestions* are more useful than questions. Rather than ask directly about emotional experience, put the request in the form of a suggestion. The therapist may say: "Pay attention to what is going on in your body [your face, gut, eyes] as you say that. Notice how you feel at this moment. Don't just rush past it, attend to it."

Sharing Observations of the Client

The therapist may also turn the person's attention to emotional experience by sharing observations about changes in the client's nonverbal behavior. The therapist's interventions may include comments on observed changes in facial expression, posture, breathing, hand gestures, and voice quality (Daldrup, Beutler, Engle, & Greenberg, 1988; Gendlin, 1978, 1996). These nonverbal changes indicate shifting emotional experiences. The therapist brings the changes to the attention of the client. For example, the therapist might say: "I'm aware that your mouth is drawn very tight as you pause between words. It seems as though part of you is trying to hold back and close off what you're saying." Or the therapist might say: "As I listen to you respond to that critical part of you, I notice that you hold your breath. You look as though you're bracing for more. Tell her what you're experiencing right now."

Such observations are offered tentatively, allowing the client to affirm or disconfirm their accuracy, as in the following examples: "I thought I sensed your body slump, as though you feel defeated and ready to give up. Did you get any sense of that?" Or, "Notice what your body wants to do right now. My sense is that you're bracing as if you're angry and getting ready for a fight. Tell the other part of you whether or not this feels true."

Developing the Language of Ownership

Clients often use language in a manner that dilutes their emotional experience. Some people use the word *it* instead of the word *I,* for example: "It makes me sad to see you not change." In such instances, the therapist may prompt the client to repeat the sentence, but this time using the word *I,* that is: "I am sad when I see you not change." This language of ownership ("I am . . ." or "I feel . . .") fosters an identification with the emotional experience. Here is a segment of a therapy session that illustrates the client's "it" language.

> "It doesn't make it any easier to accomplish what I need to accomplish [voice tight]. In fact it makes it a whole lot harder. . . . It defeats me . . . it does! It makes me not want to do anything. It doesn't make me feel good at all. It makes me unhappy when you start doing that to me."

This is an accurate paraphrasing from a therapy session. Imagine how differently the client would feel if he or she were to address the other self more directly:

> "You don't make it any easier to accomplish what I need to accomplish. In fact, I feel defeated, I do! I don't want to do anything. I don't feel good at all. I' m terribly unhappy when you start doing that to me."

In the second version, the person is more likely to be aroused enough to be assertive and to evoke a different kind of response than the Complaining Self in the first version. Emotional experience is strengthened when each self truly owns his or her experience. Some dilute their present experience by using qualifying language. To say "I feel kinda sad, sometimes, when I miss my goals in life" or "I am sort of angry with myself" is less powerful than when the qualifying words are omitted.

Developing Specifics and Details

Details can also foster emotional intensity. Clients will often talk in a generalized, vague language. In the two-chair experiment, one part of the self may say to the other part "I am upset with you." The therapist should ask for the specifics of the upset, distress, or reactions toward the other part of self. For example, a woman was talking about a recent episode in her life in vague and flat terms. The therapist's request for greater specificity sharpened her emotional response:

THERAPIST: Tell her exactly what you are upset about.

ANGRY SELF: I'm upset with you that you're still in this relationship. You have every reason to leave it, but you don't. And I'm angry that you dismissed what happened Friday at the dinner table as not worth being upset about. You were hurt by what he said to you—it does matter when he treats you badly. He scoffed at your ideas and treated you as if you had no brain. He embarrassed you in front of the children! [Resentment begins to show.]

Exaggerating

Inviting the client to exaggerate is best done when the therapist hears or sees something that appears salient, but is not being fully formed. The therapist detects the emerging expression and asks the client to exaggerate it: "Would you say that again, but in a louder voice?"; "You shook your finger at her as you spoke—would you continue to do that and do it more intensely?" Here are some additional examples of asking the client to exaggerate his or her experience:

"Your finger just jabbed the air as you spoke to her [the self in the other chair]. Do it again and do it harder . . . do it a number of times . . . good . . . keep doing it and express the feeling that goes along with doing that."

"You said something that sounded important, but you almost swallowed it as you said it. Say it again and see if you can support your words with more breath. . . . Good, see if you can say it even stronger."

Repeating

When a potentially important statement is first expressed, it is often tentative and relatively unemotional. By asking the client to repeat the statement several times, more emotion may emerge.

CLIENT: I'm sad (*slightest look of sadness around the eyes, flat voice*) that you're always pushing me to be okay [first mention of any emotion since beginning the experiment].

THERAPIST: Tell her that again.

CLIENT: I'm sad . . . (*tears begin to form, voice becomes sad*). You're always pushing for more. I don't have more to give (*pauses and tears begin to go away*).

THERAPIST: Keep talking to her. Begin several sentences with the words "I'm sad when . . . " or "I'm sad that . . . "

CLIENT: I'm sad when you push me to ignore my loneliness. I'm sad that you just want me to smile and be pleasant all the time . . . (*begins to cry*). I'm sad that you don't understand how desperate I feel most of the time.

Fostering Movement

Action tendencies are associated with emotions (e.g., shame/withdraw, anger/defend, and fear/avoid). Fostering the action tendency promotes a freer expression of the emotion. There are two ways to intervene. One is to encourage the movement associated with the action tendency. If, for example, a client says that she feels like curling up and closing out the world, the therapist could say: "Do that. Allow yourself to close your eyes and curl up in your chair and see how that feels." The second intervention is to ask that the client attempt the opposite of the current behavior. If a person becomes very still, the therapist could invite him or her to get up and slowly move about the office as he or she continues to talk. On the other hand, if movement or rapid speech on the part of the client is a way of avoiding the emerging emotional experience, the therapist asks the client to experiment with being still or quiet.

Exploring the Restraint

We are all familiar with the need to contain emotional expression at times. A parent may not want to frighten her children by showing them how upset she is. We may be very angry, but we "hold our tongues" because we might make the situation worse or even unsafe. There are times when we need to be emotionally stable now to get through a crisis and do the "falling apart" later. However, sometimes we become fixed in a pattern of emotional containment and have difficulty expressing our feelings even when it is safe and appropriate to do so.

Rather than trying to force emotional expression, the therapist accepts the process of containing emotion and turns attention to all that is involved in the containment. Often clients will notice that the emotional containment affects the body. For example, muscles and breathing become constricted, the voice may become weak and thin, posture may be compressed or rigid, or the client may feel heavy or burdened. Gently encourage the client to continue the emotional constriction but with awareness. In time, clients become aware of the burden of containing the emotion and begin to mobilize the body toward expression rather than containment.

Exploring Predictions

When a client contains emotion, it is often because of a belief or prediction that needs exploration such as "If I start to cry I won't be able to stop" or "I'll feel crazy and out of control." Explore these beliefs, predictions, and attitudes so that they are clearly understood, allowing the client to experiment with a different way of managing his or her emotions in the therapy session.

Ruth had many reasons to be angry. She was partially aware that she was angry and understood the reasons for it. However, she had great difficulty allowing herself to be angry. She became depressed, experienced heavy bouts of guilt and shame, and struggled to keep the anger at bay. She was asked to say what she believed about expressing anger. Ruth flashed on a childhood scene and described herself as being 6 or 7 years old huddled in fear in her bedroom with her baby sister. Her father, in a drunken rage, was destroying things in the home. As she reported the flashback, Ruth said: "I promised myself that I'd never allow myself to be like that. And from that day to now I haven't allowed myself to be angry." As we talked about this memory, it became clear that Ruth had developed the belief that to be angry was to be crazy, out of control and destructive. Once she remembered and understood the circumstances that led to the development of that belief, she was more willing to experiment with expressing anger in measured doses. When she found that she could express her anger without losing control or becoming destructive, Ruth was able to alter her beliefs about her anger.

In other cases, clients make predictions that are laden with fear. For example, they "just know" that if they start crying, they will not be able to stop, or that they will "fall apart," or that they will be "out of control." They make constant efforts to control the normal and natural tendency toward emotional expression, and this effort requires vigilance, leaving the client convinced that something almost catastrophic will happen if he or she relaxes his or her efforts.

There are two parts to intervention in such cases. The first is to clarify the belief or the prediction that is implicit in the emotional overcontrol. The second is to proceed with relatively small steps, so that the client doesn't experience too much emotion before he or she is prepared for it. Remind clients that they have become experts in containing emotional expression and that they can evoke their "control behaviors" if they begin to feel overwhelmed or out of control. The therapist then encourages clients to attend to the sensory experience as it happens, and to practice staying with the emerging experience for longer periods. Initial attempts may last no more than a few seconds. Each time a client makes a choice to allow emotional expression and then to control the emotional expression, he or she tends to feel more in control and to have less fear of emotional expression.

Clients may inhibit emotional expression because they do not feel safe with the therapist or in the therapeutic situation. In such instances, it is imperative that the therapist be empathic and acknowledge those feelings. Here, the therapist should not pursue further experiential work, but should instead explore the issue of safety. Only when a client feels safe and has a sense of security will the intervention be productive.

Sometimes clients will question the usefulness of emotional expression: "I've felt bad enough about this for a long time and I don't see what I'll gain if I start crying all over again." The therapist needs to explain more clearly the role that emotions play in informing the client about his or her relation with the world. We must always have a rationale for our interventions and be able to explain that rationale succinctly and clearly, while respecting the right of the client to say "No" to any of our proposed interventions.

Eliciting Emotional Responses

In the two-chair experiment, one self sometimes makes a statement that in ordinary conversation would likely evoke an emotional response. However, the client may make such evocative statements from one chair and switch to the other chair and continue the dialogue without any emotional response. When this happens, suggest to the client that he or she tells the other self how he or she feels when *spoken to* or *speaking* that way. This usually elicits feelings from one of the selves. For example: "You're pushing your point really hard. Tell her how it is for you when she doesn't seem to listen to the point you're trying to make," or "Respond to what he just said to you. Tell him what you're experiencing and feeling," or "Say how you feel toward her when she scolds and nags you that way."

Linda said that she felt "almost silly" to bring up something that seemed trivial. Someone she considered a close friend threw a party and invited her coworker, but did not invite her. She admitted that she felt hurt and then said that she never allowed herself to cry. She showed no affect as she was describing these events. She was split between a part of her that was deeply hurt and a part of her that dismissed her feelings as silly. There was a struggle between a Desired Self and a Should Self that she labeled as the Hurt Self and the Adult Self.

HURT SELF: I feel really slighted. We worked on the same production team together and I never expected to be left out. I don't know what to make of it. It makes me doubt our relationship. (*Speaks of her hurt without any affect at this point.*)

THERAPIST: Change to the other chair.

ADULT SELF: You're making too much of this. You just have to realize that the people you work with won't always be your close friends. Don't get carried away with feeling bad.

A few moments later in the dialogue:

HURT SELF: You've been too quick to ignore me and push me away when I'm feeling hurt and sad. You think that I'm always asking you to make it better. Sometimes I just need to feel what I feel and not have you get in the way of that. You don't have to do things to distract me or get me past it . . . all you have to do is acknowledge that I feel what I feel. Allow me some time.

THERAPIST: Change back.

ADULT SELF: I guess I can do that. (*Quickly adds:*) But don't wallow. I couldn't stand that. I know I try to keep you from feeling bad, and maybe I need to change that.

THERAPIST: Come back here and see if that's what you're asking for.

HURT SELF: I don't think I'm into wallowing, I just want time to feel what I feel without having to switch it off right away. If you can allow that, that's all I'm asking for.

Suggesting "Try-On" Lines

The therapist may foster the development of emotional intensity by feeding the client a sentence to "try on." The therapist shares the request with the client, accompanied by an explanation such as "I'm going to give you a sentence to say and I'd like you to experience what it's like to say it. If the sentence doesn't fit, just set it aside. If it does fit, take a moment and feel what it's like to say it." Then the therapist offers the try-on sentence—for example, "Say to the other part of self: 'I want you to love me, but all you do is criticize.'"

One client may tell the therapist that the sentence is "on target" while another may show the therapist that it does not quite fit by repeating the statement with a questioning tone or with a puzzled look. Or the client may tell the therapist that the sentence does not ring true—the therapist has missed the mark. Subsequently, the therapist and the client can search for a more accurate reflection of the client's current experience. The therapist might say, "Since that statement doesn't fit, see if you can find a statement that's a better fit for what you're experiencing."

There is a possible problem with this intervention. We have found that students learning these strategies are sometimes too eager to see a client arrive at a place where he or she feels less distress. They sometimes guide the client to that new place by feeding him or her numerous lines to say. This does not work. Clients need to struggle to find their own words and to be in that struggle for as long as it takes. This intervention has benefit only at those times when the client's experience has developed implicitly, but has not yet been expressed explicitly.

Containing Emotional Experience

There is one situation in which increased arousal is not helpful: if a person is constantly in a state of high arousal, increasing that emotional experience is not theoretically desirable. The following example concerns Marshall, who had an accident when he was in the last year of high school and is confined to a wheelchair. He identified two selves that both operated at a high level of emotional intensity. The one self exuberantly drove him to be "normal," to deny the limitations of his disability, to be accepted, and to be loved. This part engaged life in a frenetic, driven, unsustainable mode—"all or nothing." He called this self the Driver. When a letdown occurred, the other self would seize the moment. This self was unmercifully harsh and destructive, driving Marshall into depression. He termed this self the Punisher. In the previous session, Marshall had identified an emerging third part that he named the Thinker. This self offered a more reasoned and less emotional position. In the following session, we worked with all three selves, but especially supported the efforts of the Thinker, who was able to think more clearly, make better choices, and be less clouded by extreme moods than either of the other two selves.

DRIVER: (*loud voice*) Yes, for once, he and I were in agreement! Let's get him immersed in his studies so we can do this. . . . You can get him to go all out and when he fails I can kick his ass. (*Makes a spontaneous switch to the Thinker's place.*)

THINKER: And as the Thinker, I would love to say 'no' (*serious voice*). I'm not going to let it happen. Even though the two of you think you're in agreement about wanting to impress the girls, you want to impress for very different reasons. Neither are really very valid reasons. Even though yours [the Punisher] has an awful lot of appeal. He's right in the sense that you're not going to be able to keep up that kind of frantic pace (*to Driver*).

THERAPIST: You suggested that they're in agreement for very different reasons. Tell the Punisher what you believe motivates him.

THINKER: You want to humiliate.

THERAPIST: So, he's motivated by humiliation. Hmmm. Now, tell the Driver what you believe motivates him.

THINKER: The desire to be like everyone else . . . longing . . . the desire to be acknowledged . . . the thought of being loved, that kind of thing. That's what motivates him. [Clarifying the presence of a Desired Self]

THERAPIST: Uh-huh . . . Now the Punisher is looking for the opportunity to jump on him and beat him up; it's pretty clear what motivates him. You see some problem with what the Driver wants, is that right? [The therapist attempts to engage the cognitive function more.]

THINKER: Right.

THERAPIST: Talk to the Driver about that.

THINKER: I think you're wrong about wanting to be fanatical about chemistry and take it just solely on the purpose of desire—simply because you're not going to be able to impress anyone, especially if you try to impress Anna. Secondly, if you do impress her, what's she going to do? She's dating, she's engaged . . . and she's unavailable. And as for trying to find an available student, maybe, but I don't know . . . I think that it's best just to stick to your own business. Do well on your chemistry, but don't try to do it for impression. If you're *not* looking for praise and acceptance and love, then maybe you might get it. So just try and relax.

THERAPIST: Come back over here and be the Driver.

DRIVER: (*immediately excited voice*) I can't relax. I sit in that class and I listen to her speak and I see the people all around me and I want that so bad . . . they all seem . . .

THERAPIST: (*empathic voice*) What is it you want so badly?

DRIVER: To be like them. They seem almost perfect, almost god-like and I feel *so* inferior.

THERAPIST: Become the Thinker and talk to him [the Driver].

THINKER: (*deep sigh*) You're not inferior to them. They make mistakes. You'll do all right with your class . . . if you stick with your class and take a "wait and see" attitude, who knows what you might come up with. But if you take this extreme position, that is, if you drive yourself to get their praise and acceptance, then you're undoubtedly going to be disappointed.

The Thinker was beginning to be a felt presence in the dialogue, but the other selves were still not listening well to what he had to say. In this session, Marshall was intent on playing out the old routine of driving frantically to be just like anyone else and beating himself up when that failed. Over time the Thinker would have a stronger role to play in developing a less emotional struggle.

STEP 4: RESOLUTION

When clients stay with an emotionally meaningful dialogue in which there is honest give-and-take, there is a point at which the dialogue takes a turn, moves into new territory, and works toward a solution. Greenberg and his associates (Greenberg et al., 1993; Safran & Greenberg, 1991) have noticed that with "conflict splits" there is a softening of the more critical self that opens the door to negotiation and resolution. We often see a softening of the dialogue in ambivalence resolution as well. For example, Barbara, a client with depression, realized during a two-chair dialogue that the scolding and harsh part of herself was doing what her older sister had consistently done to her while they were growing up. With this new awareness and meaning, she was able to be much less severe with herself. As she became increasingly supportive of herself, her depression improved.

Expressions of Resolution

In our experience, resolution takes one of three different forms: (1) the disappearance of ambivalence, (2) the acceptance of the presence of two voices that have equal value, or (3) a decision not to change at the present time.

Absence of Ambivalence

Some clients will state that, because of the dialogue work, they are no longer experiencing separate selves but feel the emergence of a single self. They report that neither self comfortably represents their present-moment experience. This is illustrated in the following example:

CLIENT: (*to therapist, after several minutes of being engaged in the two-chair experiment*). You know, I have a sense that there aren't two of me any more. I don't think that either chair represents what I'm feeling . . . it's as if they just kinda jumped together and became one.

THERAPIST: (*checking to seek if there is a true coming together*) Fine, look around the room and decide on a new place to sit. (*Client moves to a new seat.*) Now see what it's like to talk to me from this new, unified place.

CLIENT: I don't feel that sense of struggle right now. It's as if I just know what I need to do and there isn't any part of me that wants to get in the way.

THERAPIST: Do you have any sense that one part of you overpowered the other?

CLIENT: No, it's just that we both seem to know that it's time to move ahead. I had the feeling that when the side of me that pushed so hard for change understood how scared the other side was, the difference sort of melted away.

This is an example of an *in-session* resolution. Other clients may leave the session still in a state of ambivalence, but resolve it later. One client reported that he had become compliant with a disliked but essential medical regimen; another that she found her way out of a conflicted situation with a friend; and still another that he had begun an exercise program and actually enjoyed it. In these examples, there was a shift toward change and an absence of the negative emotional reaction that was associated with the original state of ambivalence.

Agreement to Cooperate and Understand the Other

In this form of resolution a client will report that the separate selves still exist and persist in their values and beliefs. However, they have come to an accommodation where both sides are willing to listen to one another, acknowledge one another, and agree to pull together for a common goal. The rhetoric between the two sides is less harsh and more cooperative. The following excerpt concerns a student struggling to do well in high-school honors classes. She wanted to be doing much better than she was doing, but could not work up to her known capacity. Her ambivalence began as a split between her Should Self and a Defeated Self that she subsequently described as her Strong Self and her Weak Self.

WEAK SIDE: (*beginning to state clearly what she needs*) I need you to help me through this because I'm not as strong as you think I am. And I just . . . I really need your help to get through this, and you're not helping me. Can you support me and listen to me?

THERAPIST: Come back over here.

STRONG SIDE: I'm not sure how to support you. (*Then, slipping back into pressing her to "shape up."*) I know that you know how to make commitments and get the job done. Show me that you can do it for a change.

THERAPIST: Change back.

WEAK SIDE: I know that I can do it, but I need some support. You don't support me, you just beat me up.

THERAPIST: Change again.

STRONG SIDE: I don't mean to be beating you up. I thought I was supporting you . . . but I guess it doesn't feel that way to you. (*Voice begins to be less harsh.*) I guess I just have to figure out another way to help you (*Extended pause; therapist is quiet as client thinks.*) I'll hold your hand for you and be there with you—as long as you hold up your end.

THERAPIST: Move to the other chair. (*Client changes.*) Tell her whether this is what you're needing and asking for.

WEAK SIDE: That's what I want. I feel like you've thrown me out there on my own—to sink or swim. If I just feel that you haven't left me, I think I can do much better.

THERAPIST: So, when you start to feel overwhelmed and all alone, tell her what you will do to remind her of what you need.

WEAK SIDE: I need you to tell me that I can't get everything done at once. I need you to help me not to worry so much, to remind me that I'm doing pretty good—working after school and taking all the honors classes.

THERAPIST: See what she says.

STRONG SIDE: I know this semester hasn't been easy, and that it's a long time since we had some fun. I'll try to remind you that it is okay to take one thing at a time. I know that I want you to get it all done *now*, and that's not fair.

The two parts continued in this vein, clarifying what behaviors had been useful and what had not, and developing plans for how to approach school as a team effort between the two selves.

With Barbara, whose therapy is described at length in Chapter 10, signs of resolution began to occur in the fourth session of two-chair work. In the following exchange, we began with the self that has difficulty changing:

THERAPIST: Say that last part again. It sounded important.

CHANGE SELF: I guess I'll just be there for you in case what you decide to do doesn't work for you. I'll *be* there to help you through it.

THERAPIST: (*noticing emotion in her face*) Tell her what you're feeling right now.

CHANGE SELF: Terrible (*small laugh*).

THERAPIST: About yourself or about her?

CHANGE SELF: Feeling terrible about her. I'm upset with myself that I could ever do that to her.

THERAPIST: Tell her that.

CHANGE SELF: It wasn't right of me . . . I feel awful for that . . . I didn't realize . . . I'm angry with myself (*very emotional*).

THERAPIST: You're feeling a lot right now. Take your time with your feelings and then when you're ready, move to the other chair. (*After a pause she moves to the other chair.*)

NO CHANGE SELF: You shouldn't be really angry with yourself. You were doing what you thought would help.

THERAPIST: (*suggesting a sentence to say*) And I just needed to tell you that.

NO CHANGE SELF: Yeah, I just needed to let you know that what you were doing is . . . that the idea behind it [to point out all mistakes] was a good idea, but the way you were going about it just wasn't working. Just change the way you do it.

Accept the Present Situation

Occasionally it happens that clients will come to accept that they are not ready to change or no longer desire a change. The following portion of a two-chair dialogue concerns a woman with severe emphysema who was unable to quit smoking. Her doctors had thrown up their arms in frustration. She certainly knew that it would improve her health if she quit smoking, but she had not been able to do so. She said that it was time to address the issue. We pick up the dialogue after both positions (selves) have been stated.

THERAPIST: So, tell her how you feel toward her when she suggests that you give up smoking.

DON'T QUIT: I don't like you very much. You're asking that I give up the one thing I can depend on.

THERAPIST: Tell her more about the value of not giving it up. [Lending support to the side that does not get heard much in the internal dialogue. She knows all the reasons for not smoking. We know less about the side that refuses.]

DON'T QUIT: Well, I need a friend . . . and since my only close friend moved away, I'm lonely. It's been impossible to meet new friends. So . . . when I feel lonely I can always have a cigarette . . . I need something in my life that will be there for me.

THERAPIST: Any other value?

DON'T QUIT: It's comforting. It gets me started in the morning. It helps me relax when I've been worrying about my life all morning.

THERAPIST: Return to the other chair and see what she says.

QUIT: Well, like I said, I know that you get a lot of enjoyment out of it . . . but I know that it's just not good that you have a lung disease and continue to smoke. I know that you depend on it when you need comfort.

THERAPIST: (*Seeing that time is running out on the session, he shares an observation.*) So I see that each of you has something of value that you're trying to protect. You [the Quit side] are trying to look after her health, trying to help her feel physically better, and you [the Don't Quit side] are trying to keep comfort in her life and are very sad at the thought of her giving up that comfort. For homework, just continue to think about the values for each part of you, for each self. Don't try to force anything to happen. Just keep the dialogue going and pay close attention to both sides. If you want to write any thoughts down, go ahead.

At the next therapy session she reported that she had made a conscious decision to continue to smoke. She made the concession to slightly reduce the number of cigarettes that she would smoke each day, but she knew that such a reduction would not change the course of the emphysema. Weeks later she reported that this was still her plan and that she was comfortable with it.

Successful Outcome?

This case raises an interesting question: Is this a successful therapy outcome? It may be important to step back for a moment and examine what constitutes change. It is tempting to think that regarding this case change happens only if she decides to give up smoking and takes better care of her health.

To the extent that ambivalence is about changing and not changing, it sometimes occurs that clients resolve their ambivalence about change by deciding not to change or by changing only minimally. The goal of the two-chair procedure is to increase awareness and encourage intrapsychic dialogue so that thoughts, feelings, motivations, and action tendencies become available to the client. As therapists, we do not align ourselves with either of the client's selves. Such an attitude is basic to this work. We respect the client's decision to change or not to change, given that he or she has a fuller awareness of the feelings and beliefs involved in his or her struggle about change.

Early humanistic approaches believed that a full acceptance of the self "as is" opened a person to the possibility of change. For example, Arnold Beisser (1970) in a classic paper about gestalt therapy wrote about "the paradoxical theory" of change:

> Briefly stated it is this: *that change occurs when one becomes what he is, not when he tries to become what he is not.* Change does not take place through a coercive attempt by the individual or by another person to change him, but it does take place if one takes the time and effort to be what he is—to be fully invested in his current positions. By rejecting the role of change agent, we make meaningful and orderly change possible. (pp. 110–111; emphasis in original)

More recent authors have presented similar views about change. For example, Neil Jacobson (1992) wrote about couples' attempts to integrate acceptance and change. In "acceptance," the complaining partner lets go of the struggle to change the other person. "Change" refers to compromising with and accommodating a partner. Jacobson and Christensen (1998) devised three approaches to helping couples change.

The first strategy teaches the couple a different method of communication, one in which the couple learns to talk about the problem as an "it." The second strategy is to increase each person's tolerance for the other's negative behavior. The third strategy promotes acceptance by assisting each spouse in the development of self-care. Jacobson shares the view of some strategic therapists that at times the decision to stop trying to solve an issue actually makes the problem solvable when attempts to directly influence change have failed. Jacobson and his colleagues have found examples where achieving the goal of acceptance also led to actual change, although this was not always the case. Viewing acceptance as related to change is an idea also shared by Baucom and Epstein (1991), Christensen and Jacobson (2000), and Linehan (1993).

We, as cotherapists, used the two-chair approach with a middle-aged man with a weight problem. In the first two sessions the client was clearly ambivalent, with one side wanting and the other side not wanting to lose weight. At the end of four sessions, he reported no weight loss, but also stated that he felt more comfortable with and accepting of the state of being overweight. The Change Self shifted from a self-critical position ("You should lose weight") to one of marked acceptance of the way things are.

If the criterion for success was loss of weight, then this was a treatment failure. However, if the criterion for treatment success was a shift in stance of one self toward another self, then there was a shift toward self-acceptance. At a 6-month follow-up, the client reported that he had lost 40 pounds. It may be that as he backed off from demanding and directing himself to change, he was more able to change. Even if there was no weight loss at follow-up, we suggest that acceptance of the problem is a change that is positive and that lays a foundation for other positive changes. Here's another example: A woman comes to therapy saying that she wants to leave a troubled marriage. But it is possible that she can relinquish her critical position and adopt a more accepting position toward her spouse. In so doing, the accepting attitude may actually improve the marriage. Although we believe that this perspective has validity, we also believe that care must be taken so that "acceptance" is not used as a rationalization for failures in psychotherapy.

In summary, resolution is indicated by either (1) an emergence of a new position where the sides come together as a "new self," (2) an agreement that the two selves will work with rather than against each other, or (3) a decision to not make any changes at the present time.

When Not to Use the Two-Chair Approach

This approach is clearly not going to be helpful for someone who lacks basic information and understanding about what is involved in making the desired change. For example, if a person wants to lose weight but has no understanding of the necessary dietary and life-style changes needed to accomplish that goal, education, rather than the two-chair approach, is necessary. One of us (DEE) knows a dietitian who told a French fry-loving patient to stop eating them. The dietitian then found out that the patient had indeed stopped eating French fries, but was now eating deep-fried Tater Tots and hush puppies. She was not being defiant; she simply did not understand what constitutes a healthy diet.

The two-chair approach calls for the client's ability to maintain an internal moment-by-moment focus. If the client lacks the ability to maintain such a focus, he or she will not be able to follow emerging and changing emotional and cognitive experiences as they unfold in the two-chair dialogue. These clients may willingly participate, but the experiment will lack the "tight sequencing" (Polster, 1995) that is necessary for benefit.

Our experience is that people who are unable to access their emotional experience (alexithymia) do not do well in the two-chair approach or other experiential exercises. Most people do not fall into this category. However, when they do, the two-chair approach does not move them forward any more than the old, well-rehearsed lines of the debate in their heads.

Finally, as discussed above, people who are in an intense state of emotional arousal when they come to therapy may need to contain, rather than express, those emotions. Since the two-chair approach fosters the intensification of emotions, it is not appropriate in this situation. Clients who are in a state of crisis may well be ambivalent, but their decision-making ability is often extremely impaired, calling upon the therapist to assist in managing the state of crisis.

CASE ILLUSTRATION

We conclude this chapter with a case illustration that includes all the steps of the two-chair approach.

Sarah was an attractive, single, 20-year-old with a 3-year-old son. Her mother cared for her 3-year-old so that she could take classes at a community college. She had been in a 2-year relationship with a 36-year-old divorced man, Paul, whom she described as emotionally abusive. He had other relationships, disappeared for days at a time with no explanation, and stole money and lied to her. He wanted nothing to do with children. He yelled at her and demeaned her for things that were not her fault. She made several failed attempts to end the relationship, but always resumed it after a couple of weeks. Her parents and friends urged her to end the relationship. Although she knew they were right, she was unable to do so.

We met with Sarah as cotherapists, and offered her four sessions of treatment to explore the two-chair approach to her ambivalence as part of a pilot study. In the intake interview, we asked her to participate in a two-chair assessment role play, to speak first from the part of her that *wanted to change* and to respond from the other chair. Then we asked her to speak from the part of her that felt she *should change* and to respond. These simple exchanges revealed the truly ambivalent nature of her experience and were suggestive of beliefs that motivated her behavior.

WANTS TO CHANGE SELF: This relationship is an . . . an abusive relationship. You don't trust this man. You don't have the same life goals. You're very unhappy . . . have been unhappy in this relationship from the word go. There's nothing positive remaining in this relationship. You know he loves you, but love is not the issue. It's really time to close this section of your life.

RESPONSE: The only response that I can make is that there is a part of me that wants to believe him. Although my intuition, my internal self, says that he is telling lies, there is a part of me that says try to believe him. I keep thinking that maybe things will change, that maybe things will work out. You know that he does love you . . . and maybe that'll give you enough of an edge to build on for a relationship.

The Should Change and Response follows:

SHOULD CHANGE SELF: I should change because he was . . . not faithful, he lies . . . and that's not what I want from a relationship. These are . . . these are why I should change . . . these reasons.

RESPONSE: Only this . . . that he *can* change. And if you stick it out long enough, perhaps there will be a change.

In the next session, we reconfirmed the existence of her ambivalence. She said that she still saw Paul about once a week and spoke to him a couple of times a week by phone. She had challenged him about telling her the truth about other women and he told her he was not going out with anyone else. She did not know whether to believe him or not.

We described the two-chair experiment and invited her to try it. The dialogue revolved around a somewhat angry self that wanted to end the relationship and a sad self that clung to belief in Paul's love and his ability to change his ways. Here is a representative piece of dialogue from this session:

DON'T LEAVE: It's easy to set a boundary and hold to it, but if he calls . . . I go right back to it. When he does call, then I'm the one who wants to believe in him. I want to be with him and to accept him back. (*pause*) I believe that things can work out . . . that love *is* strong. And I believe it.

THERAPIST: Try saying, "I believe him."

DON'T LEAVE: Yes, I believe him.

THERAPIST: Change to the other chair.

SHOULD LEAVE: How can you believe him? You caught him in out-and-out lies before. You confronted him with his lies before. How can you believe him? Maybe he does love you . . . but love isn't the issue here. It's commitment. It's telling the truth. And he can't do it.

THERAPIST: Come back to the other chair. (*Client changes and immediately becomes very emotional.*) Just take your time. Take another long deep breath and allow yourself to feel what's there.

DON'T LEAVE: He's just not sure. You know how sometimes men can be like that. They're not sure. (*pause*) But it scares me that he's not sure. (*looking more sad*) You ask him if he might find somebody that he wants to be with. He's told you about his past, about how he's gone out with all sorts of other girls . . . and about his first wife. And I'm afraid of losing him.

THERAPIST: Say that again.

DON'T LEAVE: I'm afraid of losing him. (*Tears come for a time and then she says that she is hearing the voice from the other chair.*)

THERAPIST: Now move to the other chair.

In the following session, Sarah described the selves as the Logical Self and the Emotional Self. The Emotional Self waxed and waned, acknowledging points made by the Logical Self, but believed that if she left Paul would go on to another relationship that has all the things she wants. She predicted that she would end up feeling sorry for herself for not waiting for Paul to change. The Logical Self described feeling trapped, angry, and sad.

THERAPIST: Could you repeat what you said about staying in the relationship making you feel trapped, angry and sad?

LOGICAL SELF: Your making me stay in this relationship makes me feel angry. It makes me feel trapped. It makes me feel guilty. In fact, sometimes when I do things that I think are very innocent and nonromantic with other men . . . (*sigh*) . . . I feel sad because I feel that maybe you're passing up some potential people here by being very distant and not allowing yourself to open up.

THERAPIST: Does it feel as though she is the one who is keeping you trapped in this relationship?

LOGICAL SELF: Yeah. Yeah. You got it (*sounding more alive*).

THERAPIST: Would you tell her that?

LOGICAL SELF: I think you're the one who's making me feel this way. You make me feel trapped that I have to stay in it. You're the reason that I keep going back.

THERAPIST: Tell her what you'd like from her.

LOGICAL SELF: You're a part of my life that I need. I need your ability to trust. I need your ability to love. I need who you are. I would like for us to be able to work together and not be at such odds. I'm sure there is somebody out there that will fit both of our needs . . . not just yours, and not just mine [first overture about working cooperatively to resolve things].

THERAPIST: Change and respond.

EMOTIONAL SELF: I would like to try a little bit longer. But I'm scared. I do worry about losing my sense of myself . . . of what makes me, me. I'm scared about losing trust in people . . . and I believe in what you say. It's just very . . . I'm very scared that I'd be making a mistake by leaving right now.

There was a subtle shift from the first two-chair dialogue where the Should Self was angry and the Don't Leave Self was sad. They were both entrenched in their positions. By the end of the second dialogue there was an emerging understanding between the selves and the anger was gone. Sarah told us, before leaving the session, that she had been continuing the dialogue during the week, taking time to listen to and speak to both selves. She expressed to them that they were equally important and that she loved them both. The dialogue of the second session reflects the time she spent attending to both selves during the week. In the third session, there were remnants of fear about "being a loser" if she left the relationship and if Paul very quickly found someone else. The Stay Self acknowledged the severely flawed relationship, but protected her sense of worth by staying. She strongly predicted that she would not find anyone else. However, in the two-chair dialogue in this session, that prediction moved to the background. Sarah expressed how tired both sides were of the endless struggle. A strong desire to meet in the middle emerged, with a *bridge* being a central image. Here is a part of that dialogue:

THERAPIST: Tell her how far apart you believe the two of you are at the moment.

SHOULD LEAVE SELF: I don't think we're that far apart really. I mean we both agree with each other's truth. I don't think that we're that far apart . . . (*sigh*) it feels almost like taking someone's hand . . . I think a bridge is what I'm looking for—a meeting place in the middle of a bridge.

THERAPIST: Can you tell her what you think will happen if you meet on the bridge?

SHOULD LEAVE SELF: It's a movement together. It is to stop fighting each other from different sides of the bridge. There is a meeting point in the middle and then we can decide to go on from there.

THERAPIST: Tell her more.

SHOULD LEAVE SELF: I think the two of us together will be much stronger than both of us fighting separately. . . . I think we're both fighting to end this relationship basically. And I think we both want to do that. It's just that . . . I think we both know that would be the best.

THERAPIST: Move back to the other chair. Would you tell her if *you* feel ready to do that with her?

STAY SELF: (*long pause*) I have a feeling that I'd like to meet at the bridge, but I'd rather you do the talking. And as long as you're there to support me, then . . . I think I can do it.

THERAPIST: (*alert to the possibility of negotiation between the selves*) So, is that a proposal to her? "I'll meet you at the bridge if you do the talking."

STAY SELF: (*laughing*) Yeah. I'd meet you half-way as long as you'd be willing to do the talking and I'd know that you'd support me— even though I would be afraid.

THERAPIST: Change places . . . she's asked that you acknowledge that she's afraid.

SHOULD LEAVE SELF: I realize that you're afraid. I'm afraid too. I'm afraid maybe for a different reason. I'm afraid that if we don't end this it will be even worse and you and I would be driven even farther apart. And I don't want that to happen.

THERAPIST: How big is the gap at the moment?

SHOULD LEAVE SELF: Very small. Even the part that would do the talking still has fears. Although you think I'm the stronger of the two, I really need your support too. I'm afraid also . . . and . . . I know you know the right words, if you could help me out. (*She does not want to end the relationship with anger, but with softer words.*)

The dialogue continued with mutual support as a solid theme. The feeling of debate disappeared. The different selves were now working out how to give and receive the support needed.

In the fourth and final session, we were prepared to work with Sarah's ambivalence once more when she said that she was no longer split. She was of a single mind about what she needed to do, but she wanted to discuss with us the specifics of how to tell Paul that she was leaving. We spent the session in that discussion.

We hope that these session excerpts give the reader a sense of the two-chair procedure in practice. This case illustrates the supportive, compassionate role of the therapist. We created a place where the client could explore her struggle without judgment, criticism, or persuasion. Further, the therapist was not aligned with either side of the ambivalence. The transcripts also demonstrate Sarah's creative ability to work through the issue on her own. There were moments when Sarah cycled back through the same material, but each cycle led her to a slightly different place. There were several pivotal moments throughout these dialogues:

- Sarah revealed that she was afraid of losing her boyfriend and her *fear and sadness* were given room for expression. She had clung to her fantasy (that Paul would change) rather than endure the fear and sadness involved in letting go of him. After fully experiencing and expressing her emotions, her hope of Paul changing soon dropped away.
- Sarah's separate selves (Leave, Don't Leave) shifted from fighting with each other to an acknowledgment of needing one another.
- Sarah developed the image of a bridge and the idea of meeting in the middle. This provided her with a way to conceptualize how wide the gap between the selves was from moment to moment.
- Both selves were able to acknowledge that they were afraid. Both expressed a clear need for the strength of the other self. The mutual expression of vulnerability and appreciation helped create a meeting on the bridge.

In a 1-year follow-up, Sarah reported that within a few weeks of our last meeting she had ended the relationship with Paul. She said it took her a couple of meetings with him to do it, but that she never wavered in her resolve and she felt clear that what she was doing was right. In the interim, men had asked to date her, but she decided she was not ready for a new relationship yet. She was clear that it was "okay not to have him as part of my life."

SUMMARY

In this chapter we described the heart of the two-chair dialogue and how that dialogue can be enhanced to bring about a resolution. The importance of the development of separate selves (voices) and the engagement of the selves (contact) were stressed. We provided clinical suggestions for working with these two critical aspects of the dialogue. We described modes of good and poor contact and how to work with them. We also stressed the important role that emotion plays in the development of a therapeutic outcome, and discussed a number of interventions designed to foster the development of emotion. We addressed how the dialogue leads to resolution. Resolution occurs when the client's selves shift into a more collaborative dialogue and are more accepting of one another. Resolution takes one of three forms: (1) a new experience of "one self" where the separate selves fall away, (2) an agreement to give both selves a voice in addressing the changing needs of life, and (3) not to attempt any change. We discussed whether the decision not to change is a positive therapeutic outcome. Further, we discussed instances where the two-chair approach is not an appropriate intervention: (1) the client is either uninformed or misinformed about making a particular change; (2) the client is incapable of maintaining an internal, moment-by-moment focus; (3) the client cannot access emotional experience; and (4) the client is in a state of high emotionality and/or crisis, requiring the therapist to become active in the management of this emotionality. We concluded with an extended case example.

CHAPTER 8

Motivational Interviewing
Principles and Strategies

WHAT IS MOTIVATIONAL INTERVIEWING?

Motivational interviewing (MI) is a relatively recent entry into the psychotherapeutic scene. It was originally developed by William R. Miller and Stephen Rollnick (Miller & Rollnick, 1991, 2002) for the treatment of alcoholism and the addictions.[1] In the second edition of their book, the authors broadened the scope of MI to include any personal change endeavor, including disorders like depression and the anxiety disorders. Although MI was developed independently of the two-chair method discussed earlier in this book, the two approaches have a great deal in common. MI is an interesting integration of the client-centered therapy of Carl Rogers with the active behavior change orientation of behavior therapy and CBT.

MI and the two-chair approach share the basic assumptions of our integrative model. Both see resistance as ambivalence and as an indicator of important information about the client, and not simply as an obstacle to be overcome. They both promote the idea of the therapist working with ambivalence and helping clients to resolve their ambivalence about change, without advocating for change. The two approaches differ only in the methods that they use to deal with ambivalence and motivation.

---

[1]The interested reader can find a wealth of information on MI on Miller and Rollnick's website at *www.motivationalinterview.org*. The website contains valuable information relating to training workshops, references, assessment instruments, and new developments.

MI departs from traditional client-centered therapy because it is intentionally directive in its attempt to resolve ambivalence and increase the client's intrinsic motivation to change. It also departs from traditional behavior therapy and CBT in several ways. The most important one is the therapist's role with respect to change. In behavior therapy and CBT, the therapist clearly takes the role of an advocate for change. However, in MI, the therapist does not advocate for change. Instead, the therapist's job in MI is to help the client become his or her own advocate for change. For example, in MI, change strategies are primarily suggested by the client, with the therapist acting as a consultant for the client's change program. In this context, the therapist will usually have some input about approaches that may be helpful. However, the therapist offers proposals are proposed tentatively as input to the client, who is the final decision maker about how to approach and effect change. Finally, MI makes no assumptions about the client's readiness to change and when an action orientation may be helpful. In fact, motivation for change is a crucial target for therapy in MI. With intrinsic motivation high and ambivalence about change low, MI assumes that change will occur, with the client as the main locus of the change.

Miller and Rollnick define MI as *"a client-centered, directive method for enhancing intrinsic motivation to change by exploring and resolving ambivalence"* (2002, p. 25). Below, we consider the components of this definition.

Client-Centered

Miller and Rollnick (2002) view MI as an evolution of the client-centered therapy developed by Carl Rogers and his associates (Rogers, 1951). MI is client-centered in its focus on the concerns, experiences, and perspectives of the individual client. Miller and Rollnick write:

> Motivational interviewing does not focus on teaching new coping skills, reshaping cognitions, or excavating the past. It is quite focused on the person's present interests and concerns. Whatever discrepancies are explored and developed have to do with incongruities among aspects of the person's own experiences and values. (2002, p. 25)

In client-centered therapy, the therapist provides the conditions for growth and change by holding and communicating attitudes of accurate empathy for the client's internal frame of reference (acceptance) and unconditional positive regard. Both of these attitudes are also central to MI.

Miller and Rollnick (2002) describe MI as an attitude or "a way of being with people," rather than as a specific set of techniques administered by the therapist. The techniques are considered to implement the basic attitudes but it is the attitudes, or "spirit," of MI that are primary, with the techniques secondary. This characteristic of MI is very consistent with Rogers's client-centered therapy and with the approach presented in this book. The two-chair technique that we have discussed is only one way to implement the basic attitudes that we believe are helpful in understanding and working with resistance. MI is a kindred approach based on a similar foundation. Over time, we hope that many other strategies will develop to help clients understand and resolve ambivalence. However, we believe that a technique-oriented approach to ambivalence lacking the underlying attitudes discussed above will be relatively ineffective.

Directive

While it may seem like a paradox to describe MI as both "client-centered and directive," it is not. Although Rogers claimed not to be systematically selective in his attention to clients' statements, Truax (1966) argued that this was not the case. Truax (1966) found evidence that Rogers responded differentially to client's statements and verbally reinforced those statements consistent with the goals of client-centered therapy. MI is more explicit about this selectivity, and specifically addresses itself to increasing clients' statements relating to intrinsic motivation and resolving ambivalence about change. It is in this selectivity that MI may be considered directive.

Enhancing Intrinsic Motivation

In most therapy approaches, the therapist tries to directly influence the client to change. Although the specific change strategies vary across therapies, they nonetheless imply that the therapist adopts the stance of change advocate, explicitly or implicitly. In contrast, a major part of the job of the MI therapist is to help people increase their motivation and readiness for change to the point that they are ready to move into action. MI tries to influence motivation for change so that the client rather than the therapist remains the active agent of change.

Studies from a number of different sources emphasize the importance of intrinsic motivation and internal attributions for change. A particularly interesting study by Lepper, Greene, and Nisbett (1973) focused on children in the classroom. They first observed the children and coded what the high-rate behaviors were for each child during a free-play period. Presumably, these behaviors were intrinsically rewarding to the children. In a second phase of the study, the experimenters socially reinforced each child for engagement in their high-rate activity. Contrary to a Skinnerian prediction of increased rates of responding for behaviors followed by reinforcement, these investigators predicted that the high-rate behaviors would *decrease* when followed by social reinforcement. This is exactly what they found. Lepper et al. argued that the children's behaviors were initially intrinsically motivated, but once the experimenters reinforced the children for these behaviors, the children felt as if they were engaging in the behaviors for *extrinsic* reinforcement, that is, it seemed to them that they were doing it to please the experimenters rather than themselves.

Typically, clients who receive drug therapy maintain their gains less than those who receive psychotherapy after treatment has been discontinued. In a well-controlled experiment relevant to this point, Davison and Valins (1969) demonstrated that behavior change that was attributed to an internal source (oneself) was maintained much better than behavior change attributed to an external source. All of these studies point to an obvious but important conclusion that is relatively neglected by many therapies with the exception of humanistic-experiential ones: that behavior change needs to be based on intrinsic rather than extrinsic sources of motivation.

Exploring and Resolving Ambivalence

The MI conceptualization of resistance as ambivalence is almost identical to the one discussed earlier in this book, although the MI approach suggests some new and valuable ways of working with resistance. A "resistant" client is seen as a person who is ambivalent about change. The person's perceptions of his or her underlying reasons for change are countered by his or her perceptions of the downsides of change (e.g., fear of change, the momentum of the status quo, the benefits of the problem behaviors, fear of failing at change). Exploring and resolving this ambivalence is at the heart of MI as well as the integrative approach presented in this book.

FOUR GENERAL PRINCIPLES OF MI

Miller and Rollnick (2002) discuss four basic principles of MI. These are summarized below.

Principle 1: Express Empathy

This attitude is the same one that Carl Rogers (1951) described as "accurate empathy." The therapist seeks to understand the world through the client's own way of seeing things rather than through some external frame of reference. This is done without any judgment or criticism. It is an attempt to experience the world as the client does, and from his or her perspective. Once the therapist works from the client's perspective, his or her feelings and actions make a great deal more sense. Empathy may also be seen as "acceptance." Acceptance doesn't mean that the client's thoughts, feelings, and behaviors are somehow "acceptable," but rather that they have validity simply because they are the client's views. In this sense, acceptance is not the opposite of rejection. Instead, acceptance means placing a value on the client's experiences and way of seeing the world.

An empathic attitude accepts ambivalence about change as normal. It assumes that change may be perceived as involving risk, sacrifice, or effort, each of which could lead to a degree of avoidance of change. On the other hand, the benefits of change also lead one to approach change. Ambivalence can be seen as a form of approach–avoidance conflict (Dollard & Miller, 1950).

One of the most important ways of expressing empathy in MI is reflection. *Reflection* consists of statements by the therapist that reflect his or her attempts to understand the client's perspective. Reflective statements are more than a simple "parroting" of what the clients says. Instead, reflections are statements that *guess* at the client's meanings and experience. For example, a male client might say "My parents have been bugging me a lot this week." The therapist might respond with the statement "So, you've been pretty angry at your parents this week." The therapist's statement is just a small step beyond the client's statement and makes a reasonable guess that the client feels angry when bugged by his parents. But it's an attempt to deepen the client's experience and check the therapist's understanding of it. The use of reflection is discussed in more detail later in this chapter.

Principle 2: Develop Discrepancy

In MI, the discrepancy between our present behavior and our values and goals is an important foundation for building intrinsic motivation. Awareness of how discrepant our present behavior is with what we value and desire can stimulate motivation to change. However, if the person is unaware of how his or her behavior compares to his or her values, motivation may be weaker. In addition, if the gap between present and desired behavior is too large, motivation may decrease because the person perceives the desired goal as unattainable.

Awareness of the discrepancy between behaviors and values was a crucial factor in stopping smoking by one of us (HA). A heavy smoker for 20 years, he was quite aware of the health risks of smoking. However, that awareness did not lead to a reduction in or elimination of his smoking. One morning, he awoke from a dream that he didn't remember with the thought "I'm committing suicide by smoking, and I want to live." That thought reflected a discrepancy between his present behavior and the value he placed on living. It was this motivation that enabled him to successfully stop smoking. Awareness of either the behavior alone or the value alone might not have been as effective. Motivation for change results when the person can fully see the discrepancy between his or her current behavior and an important value. MI seeks to discover and make explicit the person's values that relate to his or her current behavior, and helps the person become aware of discrepancies between the two that can fuel motivation for change.

Principle 3: Roll with the Resistance

In both MI and the two-chair procedure, resistance to change is seen as a normal experience and an expected part of the change process. It is a valuable source of information about the client's experience, and should not be treated as an obstacle that the therapist has to break though. The blocks to change are certain beliefs or feelings of the client that make good sense within his or her frame of reference. Clients may fear trying to change and not succeeding, they may fear succeeding and thereby exposing themselves to new demands and responsibilities, or they may be apprehensive that change will make them face the unknown, while the status quo is quite predictable. They may not change because they experience themselves or others strongly advocating for them to change in a pushy and directive way. In such circumstances, reactance and the desire to maintain one's sense of freedom and control may interfere with the process of change.

In MI, resistance is a source of information about the client's beliefs, perceptions, and feelings that have to be appreciated and understood. In working with ambivalence, the MI therapist explores both the pros and the cons of change *from the client's perspective.* By conveying empathy and acceptance through reflection and other ways, the therapist helps deepen the client's understanding of the pros and cons of change, making more explicit both his or her concerns and desires relating to change. It is often a profound experience for clients when they talk about the *advantages* of having the problem and find the therapist listening and responding compassionately without dismissing these concerns or becoming an advocate for change. For example, a depressed person might state that if he or she tried to push him- or herself to become more active, he or she might not succeed, and might experience this as yet another failure that worsens his or her depression. An alcoholic might discuss the advantages of drinking that relate to helping him or her relax and reduce stress, and as an important way of socializing with his or her peers. When the therapist listens compassionately to these concerns without advocating for change, clients will feel understood and then will be more likely to verbalize their strong desires for change. In contrast, if the therapist responds to the client's concerns about change with attempts to persuade the client to change, reactance and resistance are likely to result. Sometimes, the resistance is a result of the therapist advocating for change without being aware of doing so. In such cases, a therapist shift to a more accepting attitude is essential.

If a client seems ready to change, the therapist may offer suggestions or different perspectives on change. However, this is only done either when the client asks for such input or when the therapist asks the client if he or she would like to hear these ideas. The therapist is a consultant to the client in the change process, and not the primary agent of change. If client resistance occurs at this stage, it is also likely that the client perceives the therapist as a change advocate rather than as a consultant to the client.

Principle 4: Support Self-Efficacy

An important element in motivation for change is *self-efficacy*, the client's belief that they can carry out the necessary actions and succeed in changing. One important goal of MI is to increase the client's confidence in their ability to change through the use of various strategies that are discussed below.

STRATEGIES FOR BUILDING MOTIVATION AND RESOLVING AMBIVALENCE

Strategies for Building Motivation for Change

Miller and Rollnick (2002) describe two phases of MI. In the first, the main goal is to build intrinsic motivation to change and resolve ambivalence about change. In the second, the client develops a change plan and puts it into action. In this stage, the therapist continually tries to strengthen the client's commitment to change. However, clients don't progress through these stages in a progressive linear manner. As Mahoney (1991) stated, change is "an oscillating process." Motivational problems and ambivalence are usually not one-time occurrences in therapy. Even when ambivalence appears to have been successfully resolved and the client has moved on to implementing change, motivation may weaken and ambivalence may need to become a therapeutic focus once again.

In MI, ambivalence can be understood and roughly assessed by inquiring about the *importance* of the change to the client and the degree of *confidence* that he or she can make the change if he or she decided to do so. Miller and Rollnick (2002) present two simple scales to assess each of these constructs. The 10-point scale of importance ranges from 0 (not at all important) to 10 (extremely important), and the confidence scale follows a similar form. Using these ratings, Miller and Rollnick (2002) discuss four possible combinations of these constructs that describe different groups of people.

1. *Low importance, low confidence*: People in this category are the least ready to change, see change as relatively unimportant, and have little confidence that they could successfully make the change if they tried.
2. *Low importance, high confidence*: These people are also not ready to change and they also see change as relatively unimportant. Unlike people the first group, however, they believe that they could make the change if they tried.

3. *High importance, low confidence*: People in this group place a high degree of importance on the change, making them more ready and willing to change than people in the first two groups. However, their low confidence gets in the way of their making the change.

4. *High importance, high confidence*: These people are the most ready to change, view the change as very important, and have a high degree of confidence that they can successfully make the change if they tried.

The above categorization can help the therapist determine whether work needs to be directed toward increasing importance, confidence, or both.

Basic Methods of Motivational Interviewing

Miller and Rollnick (2002) discuss five basic methods employed in MI. However, it is important again to emphasize that MI is first and foremost a set of attitudes toward people, and secondarily a set of methods. The first four methods come directly from Rogers's client-centered therapy, and include *asking open-ended questions, listening reflectively, affirming*, and *summarizing*. The fifth method, *eliciting change talk*, is intentionally directive and is specific to MI. One particularly appealing feature of MI is that its originators have developed extremely useful and specific descriptions of each of these methods. In fact, their book could readily serve as a manual of MI for studies on MI.

Asking Open-Ended Questions. In MI, the client should do most of the talking. Open-ended questions are used to achieve this goal. MI encourages the use of questions like "What are some of the things that make it difficult for you to change?" and "Can you say more about that?" Closed-ended questions (e.g., "How long did you live there?") are used only when absolutely necessary since they discourage client exploration and encourage a view of the therapist as "interrogator." Through the use of selective open-ended questions and reflections, the therapist can focus the client on those areas that seem important for working with ambivalence and change.

Listening Reflectively. Reflective listening is probably the single most important skill in MI. At times, reflection may simply be little more than repetition of what the client is saying. Used sparingly, this type of reflection can serve as a message to the client that the therapist is listening and as an encouragement to the client to continue talking. However, if a therapist uses repetition too often, the client may become uncomfortable because he or she thinks that the therapist is simply copying him or her. In addition, too much repetition by the therapist provides too little direction for the client, and the conversation will tend to wander into areas not relevant to change.

Miller and Rollnick suggest that *"the essence of a reflective listening response is that it makes a guess as to what the speaker means"* (2002, p. 69; emphasis added). People don't always clearly express what they mean. They may not be able to verbalize their true meanings because of fears, concerns, lack of awareness of what they mean, or simply not being able to find the proper words to convey their experience. Reflective listening tries to help them make their meanings more explicit and verbal.

In most other therapies apart from the humanistic-experiential ones, therapists tend to make more assumptions that they know what their clients mean. However, without exploring possible meanings with the client, therapists may well miss significant material. In the case of one of us (HA) early in his career, missing the client's meaning led to a rather embarrassing and awkward situation that was distinctly unhelpful. A 21-year-old woman stated that she sought therapy because she was having trouble sleeping with her boyfriend. Assuming that he knew what she meant, HA asked a number of questions pertaining to her sexual interactions with her boyfriend. However, it soon became embarrassingly clear that she was *not* having sexual difficulties with her boyfriend. In fact, there was no sexual activity between them that went beyond kissing and light petting. What she meant was quite literal: when the two of them lay down in a bed to take a nap, she had great difficulty falling asleep! This therapeutic faux pas occurred more than 25 years ago, but is still vivid in the therapist's mind. Needless to say, she did not return for a second session. Assuming you know what the client means without exploring that meaning can led to real difficulties in the therapeutic relationship.

There are several different ways that a therapist might use reflection, with each level listed below being deeper than the one before it:

- Repeating an element of what the speaker said.
- Rephrasing: staying close to what the speaker said with some rephrasing and use of synonyms.

- Paraphrasing: inferring the meaning of what the speaker said and reflecting it back in new words.
- Reflection of feeling: emphasizing the emotional dimension through feeling statements and metaphors.

Consider the following statement by a depressed person and how a therapist might respond with each category of reflection.

Client: "Even though nothing bad has happened this week, I've been feeling more depressed."
Repeating: "You're more depressed this week."
Rephrasing: "So your depression is worse and you don't know why."
Paraphrasing: "It's important for you to understand why your mood changes like that."
Reflection of feeling: "It's scary not to be able to understand or control your depressed feelings."

In each case, these reflections are more than simple parroting. Even repetition involves selecting an element from what the client says and repeating that element. The element that is selected is determined by the therapist's judgment about what may lead to a more productive exploration of what the client means.

Miller and Rollnick (2002) recommend the use of statements rather than questions in reflective listening. They suggest that asking questions can make the client step back from his or her experience and take an observer role in order to answer the questions. In this way, questions may interrupt the flow of client self-examination. Consider the following two identical reflections, one a question and the other a statement.

Therapist reflection (question): "Does your wife's pulling back make you angry?"
Therapist reflection (statement): "Her pulling back makes you angry."

The question reflection in the example requires the client to momentarily step back from what he is saying in order to examine if he's feeling that way or not so that he can respond to the inquiry. In contrast, the statement reflection is closer to a possible next line in the client's own thoughts. If the guess in the statement reflection was correct, the client will probably elaborate on his feelings of anger and rejection. But what if the guess is wrong? Actually, incorrect guesses can be just as helpful as correct ones, as long as they show that the therapist has been listening closely. For example, if the reflective statement "Her pulling back makes you angry" was incorrect, the client might respond with statements like:

"Not really angry, but more depressed."
"It's not her pulling back that makes me angry, it's the feeling that I can't do anything to stop it from happening."

In this way, incorrect reflective statements can also be productive as long as they reflect a reasonable guess on the part of a therapist who is listening closely to the client.

Reflections are attempts to understand and clarify aspects of the client's experience. However, therapist statements that try to put the client's experience in an external frame of reference are not reflective listening and do not have a place in MI. There are a whole host of statements that put the client's experience in an external frame of reference and have no place in reflective listening or MI. To name just a few, these include advice giving, providing solutions, persuading, criticizing, agreeing, praising, interpreting, and reassuring. Even some of the more "positive" types of statements (e.g., reassuring) have no place in MI because they involve imposing the external perspective of the therapist on the client's experience.

In their discussion of MI, Miller and Rollnick (2002) suggest that it is often useful to understate rather than to overstate when making a guess about the emotional meaning of what the client is discussing. Therapist overstatement can lead to denial and minimization of the feeling, while therapist understatement usually encourages further exploration. Reflection is selective and consistent with the goals of the therapy at that point. For example, if the client is exploring the disadvantages of the problem behaviors, reflections would selectively focus on statements consistent with them. In addition, we shall shortly see that selective attention to the category of "change talk" should always be followed by reflection or some other appropriate MI response in order to draw the client's attention to such talk.

Most therapists have learned reflective listening as part of their early training in interviewing skills and employ it to some degree in their therapy. As a result, they may consider it a simple skill that does not require much attention on their part. However, in MI it is much more than that. The majority of the MI therapist's utterances are open-ended questions and reflective guesses about the client's meaning. My (HA) experience in both learning MI and teaching it to experienced professionals is that initially it is quite difficult for therapists to use these two strategies for most of a session without also employing statements that impose an external frame of reference on the client. To see this reality for yourself, consider trying the following exercise. Recruit a student, friend, or family member and tell him or her that you'd like to talk to him or her (either about any topic or have him or her role-play a client) for 15 minutes. Use only open-ended questions and reflections. I believe this exercise makes the point that these are difficult skills to implement well, and that most therapists have drifted quite a bit away from them in their clinical work.

Affirming. In order to encourage and support the client during the change process, MI involves frequent use of affirming the client in the form of statements of appreciation or understanding. Some examples of affirmations are "I appreciate that you took a big step in coming here today"; "That's a good suggestion"; and "It seems like you're stronger than you think you are."

Summarizing. In MI, summaries play an important role throughout the sessions. Summaries not only show that the therapist has been listening, but also can be used to link material together and to emphasize certain points. Miller and Rollnick (2002) discuss three types of summaries. One is what they call a *collecting summary.* This occurs during the process of exploration and allows the therapist to collect together several themes. An example of a therapist's collecting summary with a client with panic disorder is:

> "So, the panic attacks make you feel out of control and are starting to affect your self-esteem. You're feeling that you as well as other people are beginning to see you as weak because of them. What else?"

Collecting summaries are usually short and are meant to continue the momentum of the discussion, not interrupt it. That's why they usually end with an open question like "What else?"

A second type of summary is the *linking summary* that ties together what the client is presently discussing with material discussed earlier in that session or in previous sessions. Unlike collecting summaries, which are meant to encourage the client to proceed on the track that he or she is on, linking summaries are meant to draw the client's attention to the connection between two or more previously discussed items. The following is an example of a therapist's linking summary in the case of a man who was ambivalent about telling his wife that he had had several affairs (all now concluded) throughout their marriage:

> "So, on the one hand, you're saying that disclosing the affairs to her would provide you with some relief from the burden of guilt that you carry around, and would make you feel better about yourself as a person because you were being honest. On the other hand, earlier in the session you talked about your fear that she might leave you if you tell her, and that if she did stay with you, the relationship would be strained and that she wouldn't ever get over it."

Here, the linking summary is designed to focus the client on his expressed pros and cons regarding the disclosure. In this instance, the client was encouraged to consider both sides of the ambivalence in order to help him move toward resolution.

A *transitional summary* marks a shift from one focus to another. Transitional summaries are particularly important at the end of the first session. These summaries are often introduced by a preface from the therapist that goes something like:

> "Well, we covered a lot of ground today, so let's see if we can pull it together to help see where we are and where we're going."

Transitional summaries also serve an important role in ending these sessions or at certain junctures within a session that reflect a shift in focus. For example, when a client seems to have finished talking about a particular theme, a transitional summary can be useful to consolidate what was said and to help the client move to the next step. What follows illustrates a therapist's transitional summary early in therapy with a client suffering from social anxiety disorder.

> "It seems like you've made several attempts to change your anxiety in the past. You've read several self-help books, you've tried different medications, and you've been in therapy. None of that has

helped you very much. How do you feel about what might happen in our work together?"

Eliciting Change Talk. While the four methods discussed above are basic to MI, they do not necessarily provide the client with a way out of his or her ambivalence. The fifth method, eliciting change talk, helps accomplish this. In this method, the therapist attempts to elicit change talk without becoming an advocate for change. Amrhein, Miller, Yahne, Palmer, and Fulcher (2003) found that change talk predicted outcome in therapy for drug use. They described change talk as statements reflecting commitment, desire, perceived ability, need, readiness, or reasons to change.

One strategy for eliciting change talk is *asking evocative questions.* Below are the categories of change talk that Miller and Rollnick (2002) have identified along with evocative questions to elicit that talk:

> *Disadvantages of the status quo:* "What concerns you most about being depressed?"; "How has your anxiety interfered with your life?"
>
> *Advantages of change:* "How would your life be different if you didn't have this problem?"; "What are some of the good things about losing weight?"
>
> *Optimism about change:* "What encourages you to think that you can overcome this problem?"; "What changes have you been successful at in the past?"
>
> *Intention to change:* "Is there anything you feel you can do about it at this point?"; "How important is it to you to get over this?"

A second strategy for evoking change talk is *using the Importance Ruler.* This 10-point rating of importance of change may be followed by questions like "What would it take for you to go from _____ to a higher number?"

A third strategy is *exploring the decisional balance.* Here, the client may be asked to write down and/or discuss the pros and cons of change as he or she sees them now. The therapist then explores each of these pros and cons by employing the strategies of MI including reflection and open-ended questions, moving on to other strategies like working with discrepancies between behavior and values and eliciting change talk, when appropriate.

A fourth strategy, *elaborating on a reason for change,* is a method that can highlight and reinforce this reason, as well as elicit further change talk. For example, a depressed man stated that "I know it would be good for me to get out of the house more, but I just can't get myself to do it." Several types of questions can help him elaborate on reasons for change, such as:

"How do you think getting out of the house would improve your depression?"

"Have you been able to get out of the house at all? How have you felt when you've gone out?"

The fifth strategy for eliciting change talk is *querying extremes*. Some questions that elicit the negative side of the extremes are:

"What would the rest of your life be like if you didn't make any changes in the way you relate to your husband?"

"Taking the worst-case scenario, what would your life look like if you never got out of this depression?"

Some questions that elicit the positive side of the extremes are:

"If you were totally successful in overcoming your anxiety about being around people, how would your life be different?"

"Can you describe how your life would be different if you had more control over your temper?"

The five methods discussed above are used throughout MI, but are particularly important in its early stages. For example, while eliciting and reflecting change talk are helpful, more is usually needed to help the client move toward change. In order to facilitate this movement, Miller and Rollnick (2002) discuss the importance of responding to change talk, responding to resistance, and enhancing confidence.

Strategies for Working with Change Talk, Ambivalence, and Confidence

Responding to Change Talk

Once change talk occurs, the MI therapist tries to reinforce such talk using some of the methods described above. One way of doing this is simply to ask the client to *elaborate on change talk* once it occurs. Some examples of questions that encourage elaboration are "Can you say some more about that?"; "What are some other reasons you feel it might be good to change this?"; and "What other concerns do you have about how this problem is affecting your life?"

Reflecting change talk is particularly useful here. Reflecting emotional content is particularly helpful to move change talk from a more superficial intellectual level to a more emotional level that will have a stronger impact on the client. For example, an alcoholic might flatly state that his life wouldn't be very good unless he gave up drinking. By exploring this statement through reflection and open-ended questions, it might emerge that the client is quite upset about the possible loss of his family and job, and his possible early death from alcohol-related causes.

Earlier we discussed the importance of *summarizing change talk* as a way to highlight it. Bringing together the different strands of the client's change talk may have a bigger total effect on the client then when each strand was considered separately. The therapist's act of *affirming the client's change talk* can also serve as a reinforcer to increase change talk.

These strategies point to the importance of the MI therapist's direct response to the occurrence of change talk. This usually occurs when the desired direction of change is clear, as in such problems as alcoholism, panic disorder, and depression. But when the goal is less clear, and there is ambivalence about which goal to pursue, the MI therapist adopts a more client-centered stance. The therapist's job here is not to move the client toward a particular goal, but to help the client *clarify the ambivalence* so that the client is in a better position to find his or her own resolution and make a decision. Instances where such nondirective strategies are appropriate usually involve a form of decisional ambivalence. They usually involve questions like "Should I leave my husband?"; "Should I tell my boss how really unhappy I am at work?"; and "Should I leave my job and try a new career?" Here, there is no clearly desirable option as there is in reducing anxiety or depression.

Exploring goals and values is another strategy to help clients clarify their ambivalence. The client may have explored the pros and cons of change, and may have clarified his or her ambivalence, but still not be able to move ahead to change. An exploration of how the goals of change relate to the person's values can be a way out of dilemmas such as this. Earlier, we employed the example of a man who was ambivalent about disclosing his extramarital affairs to his wife. Discussion could lead him to see that he values honesty in his relationships above all else. That would probably help him move toward disclosure. By contrast, if his dominant value involved not being hurtful to others, he might decide not to tell his wife.

Working with Ambivalence

So far, we've reviewed some basic methods of MI that are used throughout the course of therapy. These include the use of open-ended questions, reflective listening, affirming, summarizing, and eliciting change talk. We've also discussed various ways of responding to change talk in order to increase it. In this section, we try to tie all these methods together.

Markers of ambivalence may occur repeatedly throughout therapy and at different times may relate to different themes. At the outset of therapy, a client may be ambivalent about the very idea of talking with a psychotherapist. The client may be ambivalent about a particular theme that comes up in a session, about making life decisions, about remaining in therapy, and about trying out new behaviors between sessions. Ambivalence may occur in the early stages of considering change, during the process of change, and in the later stages of maintenance of change. It is a recurrent theme for most people at various points throughout their psychotherapy.

Two basic MI strategies, open-ended questions and reflections, are the foundation for working with ambivalence. For example, consider a man whose wife complains that he works too much and spends too little time with her. The man may say, "I know what she wants is reasonable, but I have trouble getting myself to work less." This statement is a classic marker of ambivalence. The MI therapist proceeds with an exploration of both sides of the ambivalence. The therapist might make a two-sided reflection like:

"So, there's a side of you that would like to please her and cut down your hours of work, and another side that wants to keep working as hard as you are."

If the client agrees and starts to talk about one side of the ambivalence—for example, why it would be good for him to cut down on work—the therapist follows his lead with reflection and open-ended questions. Often, people initially react to such an exploration with socially desirable responses that they "should" believe, but often don't believe. For example, when discussing why he wants to reduce his time at work, he may say: "Well, I can think of a number of reasons I should. Spending less time at work would make my wife happier and it's not a good way to live my life." Further exploration through open-ended questions and reflection may help him to get to reasons that are more meaningful to him.

Further, periodic summaries are also very helpful. Sometimes the new awareness that emerges from such discussions helps to tip the scale in one direction or another, but sometimes it doesn't. If the therapist believes that the client is leaning toward a good resolution of the dilemma and is almost ready to act, a helpful question is "Is there anything you want to do about the problem at this point?" The client may respond with some action that he feels ready to take, like reducing his work time, or he may say that he really doesn't know if he's ready to do anything yet. In addition, periodic estimates by the therapist of the importance of the change to the client and his or her confidence in the ability to change are often useful barometers of the client's current status regarding change.

Working with MI in the Action Stage

The majority of what has been written about MI involves preparing people to make changes by increasing their motivation and reducing their ambivalence about change. Surprisingly, relatively less has been written about working with people once they are ready to change. We believe that this is an area that deserves more attention. As Prochaska and Norcross (2004a, 2004b) and Mahoney (1991) have pointed out, stages of change are not linear and often involve movement back and forth between ambivalence and readiness. Just because someone seems ready to change at one point doesn't mean that he or she will remain in that state of readiness in the future. The therapist often has to move back and forth between stages with the client, working to increase motivation and resolve resistance at some points, and encouraging action and strengthening the commitment to action at other points. In addition, a person may be ready to change one problem, but still ambivalent about changing another.

Signs of client readiness to change include decreased markers of ambivalence, increased change talk, and an increase in statements and questions that relate to what the person can do to change. In some cases readiness translates smoothly into change, while in other cases there is still work to be done.

The MI style of encouraging action stresses the importance of a change plan that the client perceives comes primarily from him- or herself rather than from the therapist. The therapist may encourage the client to think about change with some of the following questions:

"How do you think you can make that change happen?"
"It sounds like things can't stay the way they are now. What do you think you might do?"
"What changes, if any, are you thinking of making?"
"What's the next step for you?"

These questions are followed by reflections and open-ended questions on the part of the therapist until the client has a fairly concrete plan. Miller and Rollnick (2002) make the important point that a reflective approach such as MI is not incompatible with the therapist offering advice or suggestions. The therapist has expertise and should share it with the client when appropriate. In fact, it is important in many cases to provide the client with direction for change through such interventions. The question is not whether or not advice and suggestions are offered in MI, but *how* they are offered. Below are several examples of how a therapist might add advice, suggestions, or other expertise to the interaction with the client:

"I have some thoughts about what's been helpful for other clients with a similar problem that might be helpful for you. Would you be interested in hearing them?"
"I have an idea here that may or may not be relevant. Would you like to hear it?"
"Would it be all right if I told you a concern that I have about what you're proposing to do?"

A key aspect of dealing with the action stage is for the therapist to *ask for permission* to share some ideas with the client about change strategies or to express concerns about the client's proposals. The role of the therapist is that of consultant to the client's change endeavor, rather than as the agent of change.

I (HA) have found an approach for dealing with client's between-sessions changes that is quite compatible with MI and has proven particularly useful (see Arkowitz, 2002). This involves putting the client's change plan in the context of an "experiment" from which client and therapist can both learn, rather than suggesting goal-oriented tasks to be completed by the client. With the "experiment" context, the client doesn't face the possibility of "failure" to carry out the plan, since the experiment consists of the client's commitment to *try* to execute the plan. In effect, that's the independent variable in the experiment. All the rest is data. The following is an example of how the therapist might frame the client's change attempts:

"One way that you might think about this is like an experiment. The experiment consists of your walking out of here committed to trying to make the change. Everything after that is data that we learn from. If you are able to make the change, we learn about what thoughts and feelings arise for you now that you're acting differently. If you make the change only partially, we try to find out what got in the way of your being able to do it, and we learn from your partial change. We might even learn to modify the experiment for the following week so that you can be more likely to do it. Finally, if you don't carry out any part of the change plan, even if you forget about it entirely, that's interesting data, too. It may tell us that the plan was unrealistic, even though it didn't seem that way. It may reveal concerns or fears that you have about change that we weren't aware of and that we can use to help you change in the future. The goal of the experiment is to collect data that help in your change attempts."

SUMMARY

MI is another useful method to work with ambivalence in psychotherapy. In this chapter, we reviewed some of the basic elements of MI. These include express empathy, develop discrepancy, roll with the resistance, and support self-efficacy. Through reflection, open-ended questions, and other strategies, MI helps clients clearly identify both sides of the ambivalence. The MI therapist also uses other strategies such as developing discrepancy between behavior and values and attending to change talk that help move people toward change. It is desirable to continue with the MI style even when the client is in the action stage, and ways of doing that were also discussed.

CHAPTER 9

Clinical Applications
of Motivational Interviewing

Although there have been only a few reports of the application of
MI to problems other than alcohol abuse, substance abuse, and health-
related behaviors, we believe that it holds a great deal of promise for
helping people with the problems that they typically bring to psychotherapy. MI can be thought of as "client-centered therapy (CCT) with a
twist," with the twist being the directive component aimed at increasing
intrinsic motivation. There is a large body of research supporting the
effectiveness of CCT by itself (e.g., Elliott, Greenberg, & Lietaer, 2004).
Because of the strong research base of MI in the areas of alcohol/sub-
stance abuse and health behaviors, and because of MI's focus on increasing motivation and resolving ambivalence, we believe that MI might be
an effective treatment for other clinical disorders too. However, research
support for MI in these other areas is sparse. The best designed study is
one cited earlier (Westra & Dozois, 2005) that found that an MI pretreatment significantly enhanced the outcome of CBT for anxiety disorders. There have also been a few case studies that have discussed the
extension of MI to disorders like anxiety and depression (Arkowitz &
Westra, 2004; Westra, 2005; Westra & Phoenix, 2003). Given the sparse
research base on applying MI to these other Axis I disorders, the following is presented in order to stimulate both clinical experimentation and
research on MI with other disorders.

There are a variety of ways that MI can be used in clinical practice.
These include MI as a stand-alone therapy and as a prelude to other
types of therapy, both of which have been discussed earlier. Arkowitz

173

and Westra (2004) have also discussed another use of MI in clinical practice. It involves shifting to MI during the course of another treatment in order to better address ambivalence and resistance. MI may be integrated into another therapy when the therapist resolves to use an MI style at those points in sessions that resistant ambivalence is encountered. In addition, the therapist can shift into an MI style (often sharing with the client that he or she is doing so) for a series of sessions to work on resistant ambivalence. Since MI removes the pressure for change, it might liberate individuals to explore the factors inhibiting their change.

GUIDELINES FOR USING MI[1]

In using MI for the addictions, both the overall therapeutic goals and the client behavior changes needed to accomplish them are often relatively clear and circumscribed (e.g., concerning alcohol abuse, drink less and less often, avoid situations likely to elicit drinking). However, in depression and some other disorders, the changes necessary to reduce or eliminate the symptoms are often less well defined. As a result, when therapists work with such clients, it is helpful to define two general categories with the client to guide their work: *overall distress and symptoms* and *specific changes that may reduce the distress and symptoms.* Therapists can adapt MI strategies (e.g., working with ambivalence, encouraging change talk) for use with both of these categories.

Overall Distress and Symptoms

This is the more general category that summarizes many of the client's cognitive, behavioral, and emotional difficulties. These may include symptoms like depression, social anxiety, agoraphobia, excessive drinking, relationship distress, and so on. Clients may come to therapy with these categories already in mind, or the therapist may help them develop these terms in the initial interviews.

In doing MI with depressed clients, the therapist can inquire about the advantages and disadvantages of change at this level. For example, a client might be asked to describe the advantages and disadvantages of being depressed. While clients find it easy to discuss the obvious disadvantages, they often need time and work to label the advantages because

---

[1]The following section is adapted from Arkowitz and Westra (2004). Copyright 2004 by Springer Publishing Company. Adapted by permission.

discussing the advantages of being depressed may seem odd or socially undesirable to them. Although not necessarily desirable, there are perceived advantages to being depressed for most clients, especially for those who are having great difficulty mobilizing themselves in change efforts to remediate the depression (e.g., by behavioral activation, by taking antidepressant medications).

Therapist inquiry into the advantages of being depressed must be done in a sensitive way that does not convey a message that seems critical or blaming of the client. We have found it useful to bring up this topic with depressed clients as "good reasons," seen from their perspective, that are keeping them from changing their depression. When they see the issue in this light, most depressed clients are quite able to discuss the topic. The attitude of the MI therapist is one that seems to express a sentiment like "Of course, you have good reasons for not changing. If you didn't, you would likely already have changed. If you're willing, let's try to understand what those reasons are." It can also be helpful to use externalizing language such as "What are the reasons your depression tries to tell you for staying in bed?"

Westra (2004) provides a nice example of this kind of work with a depressed client. In discussing the pros of staying the same, the client said that staying the same meant "no hassle," and elaborated as follows:

"Not changing means that no one will be pressuring me. I can't stand people always telling me I need to do things differently, be more active, stop crying. I feel so rotten, I just want to let myself be. I don't have the energy to do anything else. It's all I can do to just manage my kid's activities. I can't do anything else. I don't want to do anything else."

Specific Changes Needed

This formulation is developed collaboratively with the client to address the behaviors that he or she needs to change in order to reduce his or her overall distress and symptoms. In some cases, these may be fairly obvious. For example, in working with anxiety disorders, the overall therapeutic goal is the reduction of anxiety and the necessary client behavior changes usually focus on approach and repeated exposure. While some changes are helpful for most depressed persons (e.g., increasing activity level, changing thought patterns), there may be others that are more individual-specific (e.g., end an abusive relationship, act more assertively, seek a better job).

Many clients are also ambivalent about engaging in these depression-reducing behaviors. For example, ending a bad relationship may reduce the distress associated with it, but also may result in considerable loneliness. Acting more assertively may promote more self-esteem but also prompt more negative reactions from others. Seeking a better job may end in a better work situation or in rejection and unemployment. Often, the specific changes that the depressed client believes will help his or her depression are also perceived as having considerable risk and downsides as well. In using MI for depression, this ambivalence is explored and hopefully resolved, just as it is with overall distress and symptoms.

In this type of therapy, the therapist and the client discuss various possible strategies that might be helpful to reduce the client's depression. These discussions focus on the client's proposals as well as those that the therapist suggests as consultant to the client. These proposals might include procedures to challenge distorted thinking, efforts to increase social activity, a plan to start an exercise program, or the decision to take antidepressant medicine. When one or more specific strategies is arrived at (e.g., increasing social and physical activity levels), the therapist explores any ambivalence the client may have about engaging in those behaviors. If the client seems to be near the action stage, the therapist may, in an MI manner, develop an experiment to try out during the week. The outcomes of these experiments are discussed at the next session. Depending upon the outcome, the therapist may shift back to trying to increase the client's intrinsic motivation and resolve his or her ambivalence, may restructure the experiment, or may discuss what the client has learned from completing the experiment.

The following case illustration reflects work with ambivalence at the overall distress and symptoms level as well as at the level of changing specific behaviors to reduce depression.

Brad became seriously depressed during the year after he graduated from a technical school that prepared him for a career in computers. He found that he was no longer interested in a career in computers, and wasn't sure what other career he wanted to pursue. Brad scored at clinical levels on standardized measures of depression and anxiety. He reported significant agitation as well.

During the course of the first three sessions, I (HA) asked Brad to think of the disadvantages and advantages of being depressed (i.e., the overall level). Brad listed the many obvious disadvantages of being depressed including feeling sad, not being able to do things, having no interest in anything, and so on. We explored the possible advantages of his depression (reframed as reasons that keep him depressed) in a supportive and nonjudgmental manner. In these discussions, Brad was able to clearly identify one major factor: if his depression and anxiety improved, he would have to deal with the difficult question of what to do with his life at this point. He stated that this was one of the issues that may have precipitated the depression. In addition, if his symptoms improved, he expected that his parents would "be more on my case to get a job or do something, and I don't know what I want to do."

Ambivalence also arose for Brad in carrying out some of the between-session experiments I suggested he do, even when some of his ambivalence about changing his overall depression had decreased. Initially, the experiments centered on increasing his activity level and spending more time out of the house. In our discussion of these experiments, he reported his strong belief that doing both of these would reduce his depression. However, at the next session, he also stated that he found himself less hopeful during the week that anything would help, and that he found it difficult to make any of the changes. Rather than advocating for change, I helped Brad explore the pros and cons of engaging in these activities. Over time, our discussions resulted in his greater willingness to engage in these activities, which in turn was accompanied by a reduction in his depression. We also had to reduce the magnitude of the experiments (e.g., amount of time out of the house) to help him feel that they were more attainable for him.

In general, when the focus of treatment is defined by the client (with the therapist's assistance) as reduction of distress and as changing behaviors that may mediate this distress, the application of MI to depression and other clinical problems becomes clearer. However, case illustrations like this one may not convey the difficulties that are encountered in moment-to-moment therapeutic interactions. While the therapy with Brad went relatively smoothly, we have encountered some complexities with other depressed clients including frequent shifts in focus (either overall or specific) from one session to the next, an impatience with the more "passive" MI style for a client who was not in the action stage, and additional (and numerous) problems and foci developing over the course of treatment. An MI approach to depression is clearly a work in progress. We believe that it needs further development, but our clinical experience with this approach to date also suggests that it has considerable potential.

EXTENDED CASE EXAMPLE OF MI
FOR DEPRESSION

Rachel, a 38-year-old nursing student, sought therapy (with HA) for depression and procrastination. She had completed all of the course requirements for her degree, but was struggling with writing a major paper that was required for graduation. She felt overwhelmed by the task, and was making little headway in it.

Rachel reported three previous depressions. The first occurred when she was 9 years old and was sexually abused by a neighbor. She was unable to tell her parents about the abuse and became very depressed. She became tearful as she disclosed the abuse in therapy, but she was obviously very uncomfortable about letting these emotions show. Rachel had been in therapy twice before. She had mentioned the abuse to both therapists, but was too uncomfortable to talk about it with either of them. The second depression occurred in college and involved the breakup of a relationship with a man she had been seeing for 3 years. The depression led to her withdrawal from college since she was unable to keep up with the work. Rachel's most recent depression occurred a few years before she entered nursing school and also involved relationship problems with a boyfriend. During this time, she started on an antidepressant and reported that it had helped. However, she didn't like the side effect of emotional blunting. She also reported that she didn't like taking medication because it made her feel as if she was not in control of the situation and her emotions.

Rachel's depressed symptoms included lack of motivation, feeling overwhelmed, sometimes sleeping excessively, sometimes having difficulty falling and staying asleep, erratic eating patterns, trouble with attention and concentration, loss of interest in sex, and lack in socializing. She scored 25 on the Beck Depression Inventory (BDI), placing her in the moderate range of depression. She also exhibited a considerable amount of worry and anxiety about her progress on her paper.

Rachel repeatedly made reference to the fact that it was very important for her to feel in control, and that when she didn't, as was the case with her current depression, it made her feel "weak." When I (HA) briefly described MI as an approach that helped people find answers within themselves, she was relieved and pleased, because she felt it placed her rather than the therapist in control.

Rachel stated that for the past year she had been questioning whether she really wanted a career in nursing. She discussed her long-standing interest in art, and she noted that she had thought about pursuing a career in that field before going to nursing school. However, she felt that a career in art wasn't practical in terms of earning an income and paying her bills. Her father was a school teacher who disliked his job, but was unable to leave it because of economic concerns. Rachel said that she dreaded the possibility that she too would end up in a career that she despised and was unable to leave.

Several focal themes emerged from the first two sessions. The first level of focus was obviously her depression and distress about her paper and career. The second level, or what needed to change, involved completion of her paper and resolution of her ambivalence about her career choice. Another area that was potentially important involved her feelings about the sexual abuse, but she did not yet want to talk about it in therapy.

In the third session, we explored the pros and cons of finishing her paper. An excerpt from that session follows:

THERAPIST: When people have trouble doing something they feel they want to do, there are usually some pros and cons to doing it. Do you think this might apply to your problem in working on your paper?

CLIENT: Sure. A big pro is that it would give me a sense of accomplishment so it's not like I've wasted the last few years.

THERAPIST: So that's the big one. It would be a good feeling to know that you've completed what you've started.

CLIENT: Yeah, that's the main thing.

THERAPIST: Any other advantages to finishing your paper?

CLIENT: Yeah, I'd have a job and be earning a living. I don't want a lot of money, but at least I'd be able to pay my bills. . . . And my parents would be pleased to see me graduate with a nursing degree.

THERAPIST: A sense of accomplishment and income too.

CLIENT: Yeah, That would be nice.

THERAPIST: Any other advantages?

CLIENT: None that I can think of.

THERAPIST: What about the downside to finishing your paper?

CLIENT: Well, I don't really like nursing any more and if I finish my paper and graduate, I'm afraid I'll get stuck in a nursing career that I hate.

THERAPIST: So liking your work is very important to you, and you don't feel that you like nursing enough to keep you from ending up like your father, unhappy about your work.

CLIENT: Right.

THERAPIST: Anything else?

CLIENT: Well, I guess it delays the inevitable—getting a job as a nurse. And I also worry about being turned down for jobs.

THERAPIST: So the good news is that you'd have to go on the job market, and the bad news is that you'd have to go on the job market.

CLIENT: Yeah, exactly. I'm kind of shy. And I'm not very good at meeting new people. And I'd have to if I went job hunting.

CLIENT: So you don't like nursing very much now and you worry that you'll like it even less in the future. And not working on your paper at least keeps you off the job market and the anxieties about meeting people and the possibility of rejection. Anything else?

CLIENT: It's just easier not to do it, and the idea of attempting something and failing it is very scary. What if I put a lot of energy and work into it and it still isn't working?

THERAPIST: You would have gotten your hopes up and put in a lot and be left in the same place.

CLIENT: So it's kinda safer to not try than it would be to try.

THERAPIST: Has that been a theme in your life before?

CLIENT: I've always been an underachiever.

THERAPIST: Anything else you can think of?

CLIENT: No, those are the main things. It's the easy way out to not do it.

THERAPIST: Let me try to summarize so far and let me know if it sounds right. The main reason in favor of completing the paper and graduating is that it'll give you a sense of accomplishment, like you didn't waste all these years. Also, it would allow you to earn a living, and your parents would be pleased. The downsides of finishing is it might put you in a career you don't like, and that you'd need to go on the job market and that would face you with anxiety and the possibility of rejection. And it's safer not to try. Does that sound right?

CLIENT: Yeah. I didn't realize how many reasons there were not to finish. But I really should [finish the paper]. It doesn't make sense not to?

THERAPIST: Do you mean that the disadvantages of finishing the paper don't make sense?

CLIENT: No, I guess I mean I really *should* finish it. But I can kinda see why I'm having trouble.

Rachel began the next session by saying that she had thought some more about the pros and cons of finishing the paper and that some more advantages had occurred to her. She said, "It would be wrong not to finish up. There's not that much writing left." She tentatively thought that if she did begin to look for a nursing job and found one, it might motivate her to finish the paper. However, she still seemed fairly stuck in her work on the paper.

Since the decisional balance was not tipped clearly in the direction of change, in the next few sessions I focused on increasing Rachel's motivation for change. To accomplish this, I primarily used two MI strategies: focusing on value–behavior discrepancies and increasing change talk. Value–behavior discrepancies were emphasized by comments I made that restated her values on control, strength, and accomplishment, on the one hand, and her difficulties in completing her paper, on the other. While a part of her response to such comments was self-blame, she was also able to get beyond that and see the discrepancy. One strategy I used for increasing change talk was to have her discuss times in the past that she was having difficulties that she was able to overcome. Rachel talked about the depression she had as a college student that led to her withdrawal from college. She said that her own efforts, aided by the medication, allowed her to make a comeback and return to good standing at school. She also said that she and her boyfriend worked on their problems at the time together, and managed to mostly overcome them. I encouraged this talk, and made comments like "So perhaps you really do have the inner strength to overcome your current problems too."

We discussed her current behavior as a kind of a choice to be distressed and not write. I did this to highlight the discrepancy between her behavior and her values on choice and control. We discussed other choices including trying to write even though she was distressed, or taking time off from trying to write to reduce some of her distress. Although Rachel wasn't pleased with the choice she was currently making, she very much liked the idea that she was making a choice and that there were other choices. Once again, the importance of control became apparent. She decided not to write during the next month, but to spend her time and energy preparing job applications for next year.

By the eighth session, Rachel's depression was somewhat reduced, with her BDI score dropping from 25 to 16. She had been doing some work on her job applications. Although she said it was still difficult to work on them, she had been making progress. In this session, when she once again alluded to the sexual abuse, I asked her, as I had in previous sessions, if she wished to discuss it further. She did so for a few minutes, with great difficulty and discomfort. She provided a few more details of what had happened, and noted that she thought that it was still affecting her relationships. She revealed that she often uses sex to get men to love her and to get power over them. She reported that once she succeeds, she loses interest in sex and in the man. At the next session, Rachel reported feeling a little better during the week as a result of that discussion, but to my surprise she also said that she was "wary" about coming to this session. She said that talking about those events provided some relief, but she also feared losing emotional control if she were to discuss them further. The focus of the next few sessions was primarily on her ambivalence about talking about the abuse, and secondarily on tracking her progress on job applications and work on her paper.

We examined the pros and cons of her discussing the abuse. The results of these discussions are presented below:

Pros of discussion

"I'd probably feel better."
"My sex life might improve."
"I wouldn't feel so burdened by it."
"I know I should."

Cons of discussion

"I don't want to make a bigger issue out of it than it is."
"I don't want to dwell on it."
"I'm afraid that I'll put a lot of effort into working out my feelings about the abuse, and my sex life still won't improve."
"Maybe nothing will change if I do talk about it."

Interestingly, she used the term "should" frequently when describing reasons in favor of discussing the abuse, suggesting internally generated reactance. My impression is that her voice had a whiny "reactant" tone to it as she did.

After two further sessions spent discussing her concerns about talking about the abuse, Rachel decided to try to talk about it. At the beginning of the 11th session, she looked frightened but determined. She expressed her desire to discuss the abuse today in order to try to put feelings associated with it behind her. Over the next three sessions, she went over the abuse and the surrounding events, along with her feelings, reactions of others, and how she thought it was affecting her today. She allowed herself to feel some emotion as she did so, although after a half-minute or so of mild emotionality, she would bring it under control, repeating the cycle of emotionality and control during these sessions. By the 13th session, she reported that she felt somewhat relieved this week and didn't feel as emotional about the abuse as she had before. This session was in early December, just before the holiday season. After the session, Rachel went home to her family for a month.

We met a few weeks after she returned. At that session, she reported that her depression was much better—and she looked like that was true. Further, she stated that she was feeling better about her relationship with her boyfriend overall and also feeling better about sex. Finally, she said that she had made some headway in writing her paper. However, there were some unexpected setbacks. Her professor found some problems with how she was approaching the topic of her paper, and she had to go back to parts she had already completed and revise them considerably. Despite this, her score on the BDI was 4. We discussed her desire to end therapy at this point. She seemed determined to do so, and I asked her permission to speak with her on the phone in 6 months as a follow-up. When I did call her, she expressed her desire to come in for one session. At that session, Rachel reported continuing to do well, although some feelings of depression would come and go. Her relationship with her boyfriend was going well. In addition, she was making good progress on her paper, although it was still not completed. She reported that she wasn't feeling as overwhelmed as she had been before by the task. Finally, and perhaps most importantly, she discovered that while she didn't have any interest in clinical nursing, she did feel excited about getting a teaching position in nursing.

This case illustrates some of the core features of MI. The therapist's role was not to try to get Rachel to work more on her paper or to talk about the rape, but to increase her motivation and resolve her ambivalence about both of these areas. Rather than taking the side of change, the therapist adopted a neutral position and explored and reflected both sides of the ambivalence in order to help Rachel come to some resolution and move into the action stage.

EXTENDED CASE EXAMPLE OF MI FOR ANXIETY

This case was originally reported in Arkowitz and Westra (2004); the therapist was Henny Westra. It illustrates the use of MI with a woman who had not responded to a course of CBT for her anxiety disorders. Jill, a 34-year-old married woman with two daughters, was diagnosed with panic disorder with agoraphobia and generalized anxiety disorder. She reported chronic worry and a 2-year history of panic disorder. Her panic attacks developed about 6 months after the death of her father, with whom she was very close, who had died just a few days after being diagnosed with cancer. She had recently completed 30 sessions of individual therapy with another therapist in the community, and reported little benefit from it.

Jill participated in a group CBT program for anxiety disorders. At the completion of this program, she reported that she had benefited somewhat from learning tools to deal with her anxiety (e.g., breathing exercises), and that her mobility had increased somewhat, but that she was still significantly impaired by anxiety and panic. In particular, she reported continued and persistent worries about a number of areas including having panic attacks, loss of control, embarrassment because of anxiety/panic, and worry about her health and the health and safety of her family. Consistent with the latter, she was overprotective of family members and required continual reassurance concerning their whereabouts and well-being. In the CBT group, this excessive worry about her family had been identified as an anxiety-maintaining behavior and a target for exposures to reduce worry (e.g., she would try to reduce the frequency of her continual questioning of her children about their health and well-being). However, she was not successful in carrying out these exposures. Some of the reasons she gave were that reducing the questioning would cause anxiety and worry that she wouldn't detect things that were wrong and that it would make her feel like a reckless parent.

Jill was offered a five-session trial of MI to explore her "stuckness" and ambivalence about change (e.g., coming to the group but not carrying out the exposures). After explaining the difference in focus of MI compared to CBT (i.e., in MI, the focus will not be on making changes but on exploring your thoughts and feelings about change), the therapist proposed a decisional balance exercise. Jill was invited to identify the "good things about avoiding and worrying" and responded as follows:

> "Staying home minimizes the chance that I will be embarrassed and rejected by looking anxious."
> "Avoiding reduces my anxiety"; "Avoiding allows me to stay home, in my comfort zone."
> "No risk."
> "Worrying helps keep me from being 'blindsided' again by something terrible happening to someone I love" (i.e., repeating her experience with her father's sudden death).
> "Being overprotective allows me to keep my children and husband safe."
> "Worrying gives me a sense of control."

During this exercise, the therapist helped Jill elaborate and validate each of the advantages of the status quo, primarily using reflection and open-ended questions. For example, Jill responded that the greatest incentive for her worrying was to protect her from being caught off-guard by the sudden illness of herself or someone in her family. When the therapist inquired why this was so important, Jill began to tearfully discuss the loss of her father and the difficulties she still experienced in adjusting to his absence. She described how her father had been a highly supportive presence for her and that the loss left her with an even greater resolve to ensure that unpredicted, sudden illness would not befall her or her family. Jill explained that relinquishing the hypervigilance and preparedness for illness/death that her worrying provided would make her feel even more vulnerable and afraid than she felt at present.

The role of the MI therapist here was simply to explore and elaborate the obstacles to change in order to validate and affirm them from the client's perspective. For example, in this case the therapist responded with comments like "I'm beginning to understand why you would have difficulty stopping the worry. By worrying, you feel that you're doing the best you can to prevent a repeat performance of what you went through with your father's death."

Following elaboration of the "good things" about avoidance and worry, Jill was invited to elaborate the "not so good things." These included:

"Avoiding makes me more anxious."

"I feel out of control because I can't stop worrying."

"Worrying puts limits on my family—for example, they can't travel."

"I worry that my family will get sick of my anxiety and eventually reject me."

"It's exhausting."

"I hate modeling worry for my daughters."

"I'm not the adventurous person I long to be and once was."

Jill tearfully described the negative impact of her anxiety and avoidance on her family. The therapist encouraged her to think about what her life would be like in an ideal world without the anxiety. In response, Jill said that in this scenario she would have more freedom and spontaneity, and that she would feel more like her old adventurous and outgoing self.

The therapist also worked to help Jill resolve her ambivalence about change by indirectly trying to help tip the scales of the decisional balance toward change. For example, Jill was invited to participate in a role play where the therapist articulated the pros of the status quo and she articulated the arguments for change. In addition, she accepted an invitation to write two letters, one envisioning her future under conditions of relinquishing her anxiety and the other under conditions of her anxiety persisting. The therapist also helped Jill to develop discrepancy between her current behaviors and values. For example, the therapist stated: "It seems that worrying gives you a sense of control. Yet you also feel out of control when you worry. Can you help me understand that?" and "How is it that someone who values freedom and adventure so much ends up staying home most of the time?"

During the course of these sessions, Jill decided to take time to more actively grieve her father's death. For the first time in 2 years, she had taken out and read the condolence cards she had received after her father's death. She also wrote a long letter to her father describing how she missed him; spent more time reminiscing about her father with her husband; and made plans to visit her father's grave. Although she was highly tearful in relaying these developments, she reported a profound sense of relief—"like a weight is being lifted off my shoulders." She also noted making active plans for exposure exercises such as purchasing tickets to a play outside of the city that she and her husband were eager to see, making plans to visit friends overnight in another city, and taking her children to an aquatic park in another city.

By the fourth session of MI, Jill had moved to the preparation stage of change as reflected in this statement:

"I know it's going to be hard but I'm ready to do the things I've been avoiding. The timing is good. I know I have to do them and I have the support of my family to help me get through. I think I even know what I need to do. I just need some support to help me follow through."

When clients shift into the preparation stage, it is important for therapists to shift the focus of treatment accordingly from the use of reflective ambivalence resolution strategies to more active planning for change.

The final session of MI was devoted to assisting Jill with developing a realistic change plan. Consistent with the client-centered, evocative nature of MI, Jill's expertise and ideas were first enlisted through inquiries such as "What exactly do you see yourself as needing to do to overcome your anxiety?" and "Walk me through step by step, what you intend to do to move past your anxiety." This yielded many concrete ideas from Jill including adaptive self-talk and graded exposure exercises. The therapist's role in the preparation stage is to enhance commitment to and optimism about the change plan (e.g., "What qualities do you possess, or what previous experiences have you had, that tell you that you could make this work?") and to offer any additional suggestions/ guidance that may contribute to the success of the client's plan. The therapist asked Jill whether she might like to hear some supplemental ideas based on the therapist's experience regarding what had been helpful to others in overcoming worry and panic. When she responded affirmatively, the therapist described interoceptive exposure and worry exposure and enlisted Jill's reactions to these suggestions. Jill expressed some reluctance (which was managed with simple reflection: for example, "Yes, it does sound like it might make things worse. Most people have that same reaction.") and then was invited to consider the pros and cons of these strategies. Importantly, such processing is done in a "take it or leave it" style in MI.

By the final MI session, Jill appeared visibly brighter in affect. She announced that she was beginning to more actively engage in exposure activities (e.g., taking her daughters to the aquatic park outside the city, resisting the tendency to go to the doctor when she had "unusual" pains) and she reported that she was having much greater success in doing these exercises. She described increasing resolve to "get rid of" the anxiety and increasing awareness of and intolerance for the negative impact of her anxiety on her and her family's functioning. After completion of the five MI sessions, Jill was seen for three additional sessions focused on carrying out various CBT strategies for her anxiety and worry. Standardized primary outcome measures (e.g., Penn State Worry Questionnaire, Agoraphobic Subscale of the Fear Questionnaire) reflected considerable change to the normal range from after the group CBT to after the eight MI sessions. In reflecting on what was helpful to her in the sessions, Jill noted, "I feel like I finally understand why I couldn't get over my anxiety before. I always had a sense of what I needed to do for my anxiety but now I feel more confident that I can and will do it."

SUMMARY

In using MI for many problems other than addictions, the focal problem is often general distress, for example, depression and generalized anxiety, rather than a focal behavior pattern like drinking or drug use. For this reason, it is necessary to define a focus so that the therapist can work with ambivalence and change. In this chapter we proposed a two-level approach to develop such a focus. The first level is overall distress. The second level consists of the changes needed to reduce the overall distress. The MI therapist works with both of these levels using the principles and strategies of MI. Several clinical cases were presented to illustrate the application of MI to depression and anxiety.

CHAPTER 10

Integrating Ambivalence Work with Other Therapeutic Approaches

There is an influential movement in the field of psychotherapy known as "psychotherapy integration" (see Arkowitz, 1997, 2002; Norcross & Goldfried, 1992). This movement emphasizes common factors across different therapies, as well as the matching of specific treatments to specific people and specific problems. Different strategies for integration have been examined (Arkowitz, 1997). Two of these, combination and integration, have received considerable attention. In this chapter, we consider both of these as ways that ambivalence work can be used with other therapies. Some of the main ways that ambivalence work can be used in clinical practice are:

- As a *stand-alone* treatment.
- *Combined* with other types of therapy.
- *Integrated* with other types of therapy.

AMBIVALENCE WORK AS A STAND-ALONE TREATMENT

Both MI and the two-chair approach can and have been used as the primary therapy. MI is a relatively complete therapy that includes therapy strategies and ways of relating to clients as they move from low motivation through resolving their ambivalence and toward making change. Chapter 8 described the use of MI as a stand-alone therapy.

Two-chair work has more often been used in the context of a broader humanistic therapy (e.g., gestalt therapy or the process-experiential therapy of Greenberg et al., 1993), along with other strategies. However, it can also be used as a brief stand-alone treatment for certain people and problems (see Arkowitz & Engle, 1995). Of course, any responsible therapist should include a thorough evaluation of the person and his or her problems before proceeding with any treatment. If the therapist determines that the problem centers around ambivalence, he or she may find it appropriate to primarily employ ambivalence work. In such cases, the assumption is identical to that of MI, that is, that resolving ambivalence concerning change will lead to significant changes. We have found that people with more focal ambivalence problems can benefit from just a few sessions of two-chair work, while for others it may need to be followed up by further two-chair sessions and/or some other treatment approach.

In many instances, people seek therapy for a problem that directly relates to ambivalence. Often, the client describes the problem as "I don't know whether to do X or Y"; or "I know what I need to do, but I just can't get myself to do it." We have encountered numerous clinical problems that fit these kinds of descriptions, including:

- Addictive behaviors (e.g., alcoholism and drug use).
- Lifestyle behaviors (e.g., exercise, diet, and weight loss).
- Compliance with a medical regimen (e.g., for diabetes, hypertension, or dialysis treatment).
- Stress reduction (e.g., decreasing work time and increasing relaxation time).
- Significant life decisions (e.g., committing to a relationship; ending a relationship, changing jobs or careers, having a child, relocating).
- Changing problematic interpersonal behaviors (e.g., excessive anger, lack of assertiveness, excessive dependency, emotional distance in close relationships).

Once the ambivalence has been clearly identified, the therapist may initiate two-chair work as described in Chapters 5–7.

USING AMBIVALENCE WORK
WITH OTHER THERAPIES

General Considerations

Our experience in using ambivalence work with other therapies has primarily involved humanist therapies and CBT. The approach is entirely congruent with most humanistic approaches, and is in fact derived from that point of view.

Ambivalence Work and CBT

Our experiences with ambivalence work used with CBT have been quite positive. Many of the cases cited throughout this book have come from work of this type. The extended case at the end of this chapter is a further illustration of such a combination. One of us (HA) is an experienced CBT therapist and has used both a combination and an integration of CBT and ambivalence work for many years. One reason that he has found it so easy to move back and forth between CBT and ambivalence work is that the relationship he forms with clients for CBT has many of the characteristics of the "MI spirit." His stance is not directive or overly didactic. Instead, he places emphasis on the idea of the client as the agent of his or her own change and the therapist as a consultant to this endeavor. In such a relationship context, moving back and forth between CBT and ambivalence work is smooth. However, when the CBT occurs in the context of a more directive and didactic therapist style, the client may note the difference. A little later in this chapter, we present a way that the therapist might introduce ambivalence work into another therapy that we have found useful for introducing ambivalence work into CBT and other therapies.

Ambivalence Work and Psychoanalytic Therapies

Neither author is an expert in either psychoanalytic or family systems approaches to psychotherapy. One of us (HA) has had a moderate amount of training and experience in psychoanalytic therapies, but they are neither his main nor his preferred approach to therapy. As a result, we are not able to speak with authority or experience in using ambivalence work in either psychoanalytic or family therapies.

It appears that ambivalence work is incompatible with orthodox Freudian psychoanalysis. While we believe that the "MI spirit" can be useful in any therapy, including psychoanalysis and psychoanalytic therapy, we recognize that Freudian psychoanalysis has its own well-delineated way of working with ambivalence and resistance in psychotherapy. Our approach is potentially more compatible with more modern relational and object relations psychoanalytic therapies, as discussed in Chapter 2.

A large percentage of practicing therapists describe themselves as "eclectic" (Norcross & Prochaska, 1988). Many work from a base of psychoanalytic theory and treatment, but also incorporate ways of thinking about and working with people from other therapies. We believe that such therapists can easily incorporate ambivalence work into their treatment.

Ambivalence Work and Noncompliance in Medical Treatments

Although our focus has been on working with resistant ambivalence in psychotherapy, we believe that our approach has great potential for working with noncompliance too. In Chapter 1, we reviewed some data on the disturbing prevalence of noncompliance. While the use of ambivalence work in health care could easily constitute the subject of another book, we wish only to emphasize here that the ideas that we have proposed for psychotherapy also have great potential for compliance in medical care. Some beginnings in this direction have already been made (e.g., Botelho, 2004; Resnicow et al., 2002; Rollnick, Mason, & Butler, 1999). However, we are unaware of any applications of the two-chair method to medical noncompliance.

Most physicians give their advice and suggestions in a fairly directive manner rather than in the more supportive MI style discussed in this book. In fact, the directive style may be one reason for the high prevalence of noncompliance. While few physicians would likely use either MI or two-chair work in a formal manner, they may benefit from learning the less directive method of presenting recommendations to patients in the manner that we have discussed.

One way that ambivalence work can be used with noncompliant medical patients is to have a psychologist work with the patients as a prelude to or along with the medical treatment by the physician. In one possible scenario, the physician could refer such patients to a psychologist for brief ambivalence work during the patient's treatment. Since even brief MI has been shown to have an impact, such treatment need not be prolonged. Using ambivalence work for noncompliance with medical regimens has a great deal of potential, but research is needed to see if that potential can be fulfilled.

Combining Ambivalence Work with Other Therapies

The combination approach is basically an additive one. The therapist adds ambivalence work to the existing therapy either by devoting several whole sessions to ambivalence work or by devoting parts of some sessions to that work. In the combination format, ambivalence work and the rest of the therapy are rather distinct, with each having a relatively clear beginning and ending. The ambivalence work may be conducted by the same therapist who does the other treatment or by a different therapist. While ambivalence work has usually been used as a prelude to another treatment, it can also be employed during the course of another therapy.

Ambivalence Work as a Prelude to Other Therapies

If ambivalence work can increase motivation for change, it certainly makes sense to consider its use as a pretreatment for other types of therapy. Both the two-chair approach and MI can be used in this manner. In this sense, ambivalence work is rather unique. To our knowledge, there has been only one attempt to use a pretreatment to enhance the effects of a subsequent therapy. Jerome Frank (1978) and his colleagues developed and researched a psychoeducational preparation for therapy. In their intervention, the interviewer explained to the client what he or she could expect to occur during the therapy, provided a rationale for the therapy, and tried to generate positive expectations about improvement. Several studies demonstrated that subjects who received this intervention had greater therapeutic improvements on several measures compared to controls (Frank, 1978). Only a few studies on therapy preparation appeared until the early 1990s when interest in treatment preparation was stimulated by the emergence of MI. As yet, we know of no instance in which two-chair work has been used as a prelude to other treatments, but its similarity to MI suggests that it might work equally well. Research on the effectiveness of MI as a prelude to therapy was reviewed in Chapter 5.

The prelude of either MI or two-chair work may be done by the therapist who will be doing the subsequent therapy or by a different therapist. It's interesting to note that MI as a prelude has enhanced the efficacy of even highly directive subsequent treatments like those based on a 12-step model. At present, there is no data to guide the clinician in deciding whether the therapist who does the pretreatment should be the same or different from the one who does the subsequent treatment

Ambivalence Work Added during the Course of Other Types of Therapy

A "piece" of ambivalence work can be added to the treatment during the course of therapy with another approach. In this type of combination, the therapist and the client first identify markers of ambivalence relating to one of the client's problems. If the therapist thinks that either MI or the two-chair approach might help in the exploration or resolution of the ambivalence, the therapist can introduce the possibility of such work as an "experiment." The reader is referred to Chapter 5 for suggestions on introducing the two-chair experiment. MI can be introduced in various ways. One of us (HA) has used an introduction that goes something like the following:

> "Now that we're exploring your ambivalence about _____,
> I'd like to introduce one way of working with it that might be
> helpful. In this approach, which is called motivational interviewing,
> I become more like a mirror to your comments, reflecting them,
> but also trying to add meaning as I reflect them to you. It may seem
> a little different from the way we usually interact, but it shouldn't be
> that different. The purpose of this approach is to help you see more
> clearly and understand more deeply both sides of your ambivalence.
> Hopefully, this will be helpful in resolving the ambivalence as well.
> Would you like to try it for a few minutes?"

After a period of time of working in this way, the therapist may ask the client for feedback about his or her experience with the ambivalence work, and ask if he or she would like to continue to use it in this session or others.

Integrating Ambivalence Work with Other Therapies

The integrative approach is more seamless (Wachtel, 1991) than a simple combination. In it, the therapist moves naturally to examining and working with ambivalence as it arises in the course of another therapy.

Using MI or the two-chair approach can bring to light material about ambivalence that can inform work in the other therapy, or these interventions can be used to work directly with ambivalence that arises in the course of the other work. Here we are describing what Messer (1992) has called "assimilative integration" in which the therapist works primarily from one theoretical approach, but integrates aspects of other therapies into that base. Ambivalence work integrated with other therapies can be particularly useful in eliciting core beliefs that can subsequently be worked on with either approach. Ambivalence work is certainly useful when combined or integrated with CBT. In CBT, clients are usually given therapy-related homework assignments to carry out during the week. Several studies have shown that the greater client compliance is with these assignments, the better the outcome of the therapy (Detweiler & Whisman, 1999). Nonetheless, noncompliance is a significant problem for CBT, and there is good reason to believe that greater compliance would enhance treatment outcome.

However, the stance taken by the therapist in ambivalence work differs from the stance taken by some cognitive-behavioral therapists. Although Beck et al. (1979) describe the relationship context of CBT as "collaborative empiricism," many cognitive-behavioral therapists become less collaborative and more directive when it comes to homework (see Newman, 2002). In fact, the very term "homework" implies a teacher who gives a student work to do, with the implicit understanding that the teacher will be pleased if the work is done and displeased if it is not done. We believe that while such attitudes may not be directly expressed by CBT therapists, it colors the way many therapists conduct CBT. The therapist becomes invested in the client completing the homework, and usually takes a stance that advocates for change. This may work well for many nonreactant people, but, as we discussed earlier, such advocacy of change by the therapist may elicit resistance and noncompliance in many clients.

One of us (HA) is a trained and experienced cognitive-behavioral therapist who has published in the area and coauthored the *Comprehensive Handbook of Cognitive Therapy* (Freeman, Simon, Beutler, & Arkowitz, 1989). However, even before he discovered MI, he used "homework assignments" in a way that is consistent with the approach taken in this book (Arkowitz, 2002). He does not use the words "homework assignments" when introducing the possibility of between-session activities to the client. Instead, he proposes the possibility of an "experiment" that the client might wish to try. It is clearly left to the client to agree to try it or not—but the majority do try. The client is also invited to modify the experiment proposed by the therapist, or even to come up with his or her own experiment. The therapist tells the client that whatever occurs, it's likely to provide useful information, even if the client forgets to do the experiment. Such an outcome might reveal that the experiment was more difficult or anxiety-arousing than the therapist previously thought. If the client thought about carrying out the experiment but didn't, the therapist can inquire about the thoughts and feelings that occurred when he or she was considering trying the experiment. Of course, if the client completed the experiment, the discussion focuses on what he or she learned from it. In this way, the therapist is not seen as the "task master" or advocate for the client carrying out the experiment, thereby minimizing potential reactance and noncompliance.

Combining MI and Two-Chair Work

Although both MI and two-chair work are based on similar relationship stances and underlying rationales, they are rather different procedures. In our experience with both, we have found that a small percentage of people may have difficulty with two-chair work once it is explained to them, usually because they are worrying about their "performance" and stage fright. For such individuals, and also for those who are in crisis, MI may be the more appropriate choice. However, assuming that the client is open to both procedures, we believe that they may usefully complement each other, and that each of them can make some unique contributions to understanding and working with ambivalence.

The basic format for working with ambivalence in MI is "Reasons for Change" and "Reasons Not to Change." Exploring both sides of the ambivalence usually reveals fears, desires, and conflicts beyond the superficial socially desirable reasons. The basic format for the two-chair method is "The Side That Wants to Change" and "The Side That Struggles against Change." These two strategies don't necessarily lead to the same places, but they might both be useful ways to work on ambivalence.

In MI, people usually remain focused on the pros and cons of change and explore them more deeply with the assistance of the therapist. While MI may reveal information about emotions, and while clients may experience emotion during this exploration, it is our impression that experiencing emotion during the course of two-chair work is much more common, is to be expected (according to the theory under-

lying the approach), and is often quite intense. Thus, one major difference we have observed between the two approaches is that two-chair
work is usually more emotional than MI. Along with Greenberg et al.
(1993), we believe that people may reveal more about their underlying
schemas while they are experiencing relevant emotions than they may
during a less emotional procedure. The role of emotion in understanding and working with ambivalence has not yet been clarified by any
research. We know that many studies support the effectiveness of MI for
resolving ambivalence, but we also wonder whether MI might not be
even more effective if greater emotional experiencing occurred during
the process. If so, this would support the use of a combination of MI and
two-chair work.

Another difference we have noted is in the type of information
elicited by each of these two approaches. MI elicits reasons for and
against change. These reasons are not just the superficial socially desirable ones that people initially report, but move toward the deeper and
more basic reasons that are subjectively important to the individual. The
two-chair approach elicits more complex "schemas" when splits are
explored. These may include the ones discussed earlier in the book—for
example, the Should Self and the Reactant Self, and the Desired Self and
the Fearful Self. Schemas contain more information than reasons, and
include cognitive, behavioral, and action components.

Two-chair work is more fluid and evolving than MI. For exam-
ple, the initial split is rarely the one that is relevant for the client later
in subsequent sessions, or even later in the same session. The "occu-
pants" of each chair typically evolve and change. For example, a client
may start with a critical "Should" side that later evolves into his or
her father and then into other authority figures in his or her life. The
"Reactant" side may start as stubborn and oppositional, but may
evolve into a younger, fearful, child-like side that the client might
identify as the "child" in him or her. Further evolutions may occur as
the work proceeds. While there is also some similar evolution in
MI—that is, the client's initial reasons for change may not be the ones
with which the client ends—there is less fluidity in the MI process.
The research literature is unable to tell us if these differences favor
one or the other approach. Our only point here is that they are rather
different procedures and take clients through somewhat different processes even though their goals are similar. Clinicians may find it useful
to move between MI and two-chair work to learn from the different
types of information that may emerge.

Finally, we have found that it is somewhat more difficult and takes longer to train therapists in the two-chair approach than in MI. This may be because two-chair work is much different than the usual clinical interaction, while MI more closely resembles what many clinicians already do.

A PILOT STUDY ON INTEGRATING AMBIVALENCE WORK AND CBT

Several years ago, the authors conducted a pilot study on the effects of an integrated short-term treatment involving two-chair ambivalence work and CBT (Arkowitz & Engle, 1995) for people who were ambivalent about making some important life changes. We advertised in a university staff newspaper, looking for people who were trying to make a significant change in their lives and having trouble doing so. Our advertisement mentioned an "experiment" in which we offered to work with people for six half-hour sessions at no charge, taking measures before and after treatment, and at follow-up when possible. Those who responded presented with an array of problems like obesity, cigarette smoking, depression, and ambivalence about staying or leaving an intimate relationship.

In the first session, after some general introductory exchanges, we presented each client with the model that ambivalence is a normal state of affairs, and that our goal was to help identify the sources of the ambivalence so that he or she could decide what he or she wanted to do about the change he or she wished to make. We invited each client into a two-chair experiment as described earlier in this book. The initial experiment involved the side that wanted to make the change and the side that "struggled against" the change. All the clients found this way of looking at their dilemma compatible. We proceeded to a two-chair interaction between those two sides. Following about 10 minutes of this two-chair work, we discussed the experiment with the client. This discussion often centered on dysfunctional beliefs that emerged during the two-chair work. A CBT approach was used to work on those beliefs in the rest of the session. Subsequent sessions followed the same format of a few minutes of open-ended discussion or inquiry regarding any between-sessions experiments, approximately 10 minutes of two-chair work, some time devoted to discussing the results of the two-chair work, and the remaining time was spent on CBT.

Even in a six-session treatment of this kind, approximately six of the nine people showed demonstrable positive changes (e.g., weight loss, reduction in smoking, reduction in depression, deciding that a current romantic relationship was not a healthy one and leaving it).

We are not presenting these cases as evidence of the effectiveness of the integrated approach, but more as an illustration of it. The participants were not seeking psychotherapy, but instead volunteered for an experiment that might be useful to them. Further, this report was simply a series of case studies with measurement and not a controlled outcome study. Next, we present one of these cases in some detail to illustrate the integration of two-chair work and CBT.

CASE EXAMPLE OF AN INTEGRATION OF TWO-CHAIR AMBIVALENCE WORK AND CBT

Barbara was a 24-year-old graduate student in economics who had sought therapy from the campus mental health clinic. She was referred to us at the university psychology clinic because of a depression that extended back to her last year of college. She had had a 10-pound weight gain that she had reversed just before beginning treatment. She suffered from hypersomnia with some initial insomnia, fatigue, suicidal ideation, depressed mood, loss of interest or pleasure, and difficulty in thinking and concentrating. Her grade point average had fallen considerably. She had no history of suicide attempts. Her BDI score at the time of the first session was 23, which confirms the presence of a moderate degree of clinical depression.

Barbara also reported that over the past few months she had been withdrawing from people. Death had claimed her best friend when she was in grammar school, and more recently her college roommate. As a result of these significant losses, she was hesitant to get close to people. She had been deeply hurt by friends in the past, and currently had been hurt by her friends at church. She had broken off a relationship with a boyfriend shortly before seeking treatment.

Assessment and Session 1

An initial diagnostic interview revealed that she fit the criteria for major depression, as well as for dysthymic disorder. Two of our assessment procedures were designed to access self-schemas that may be related to change: the Selves Questionnaire and a performance measure (a two-chair assessment procedure).

The Selves Questionnaire asked for Barbara's responses to various aspects of self (i.e., self-schemas) including Actual Self, Desired Self, Should Self, Feared Self, Can Self, and Expected Self. As discussed earlier, we were particularly interested in the mismatches or nonmatches (both of which imply ambivalence compared to the matches).

Next, we asked Barbara to participate in the two-chair assessment procedure. We began by suggesting that most people who are trying to change have a side of themselves that wants to change and a side of themselves that struggles against change. We told her that we wanted to get to know both sides of her. From the chair in which she was sitting, she was asked to face an empty chair and speak from the "side of you that really wants to change your depression."

Barbara responded:

> "I'm the type of person that likes to accomplish things and not get down . . . not let them get me down. I like to make others happy and that makes me happy. [Voice changes to slight whine.] I don't know. I just, I like things, I want things to go better and not worry so much."

When prompted to say something about her affective state, she said that this side felt:

> "I am impatient to change. I feel very anxious, almost impatient, 'cause I want it [change] so badly. I know it takes time, but I'm very impatient about it."

Next, we asked her to sit in the other chair and to "be the side of yourself that struggles against changing your depression." From this perspective, she said:

> "Okay, I'm the person that does not like change. I don't *want* to change. I have a hard time with change. [When] things don't go the way I have them set, I have a hard time getting over it. If somebody comes in and interrupts my way of life . . . I get irritated and annoyed and . . . I just don't like to go along with it. I like things to go *my* way. I'm very stubborn about that. . . . I just don't like the feeling of something changing on me. I like to be safe and secure."

When asked about the emotions on this side, she said that to change is look forward to a whole different way of life and said, "It's scary." When she responded from the "No Change" side, there were hints of an oppositional or reactant self who can be stubborn and react with irritation to demands for change. This foreshadowed material that evolved over the next few sessions.

Barbara was also requested to speak from the part of her that "should" change and the part that reacts to the "should" self. The "Should" side suggested that she should change because she was making others miserable. She responded from the other chair that she did not like having any kind of expectation placed on her.

After these initial assessment exercises, we moved on to a general discussion that led to the development of some of the themes that we pursued in therapy. Barbara reported that she did not want a romantic relationship with anyone until she could depend on herself. While she was discussing her friends in graduate school, information about Barbara's automatic thinking and self-image emerged. She felt inferior to her friends. We worked with her to change this belief into a hypothesis to be examined rather than a conclusion to be automatically accepted. She agreed, and we proceeded to examine confirming and disconfirming evidence related to this belief.

We explored her relationships and feelings about closeness, and Barbara revealed that "I want close friends, but I don't want to let them in. I don't want to have to let people know who I am." She seemed afraid that if she let herself get close to people she would be rejected and hurt. But keeping her distance from people seemed to make her more depressed. After we recast these beliefs as cognitive-behavioral hypotheses, she agreed to treat them as such during the coming week.

We shared with Barbara our observations about her ambivalence and she said that our observations were accurate: part of her wanted to move toward people, and part of her seemed afraid to do so. She reported that she felt less depressed when she was with people. The fear of getting hurt again, however, had recently kept her away from people, increasing her depression. We explained the two-chair approach. With her agreement, we moved into the experiment.

She began to engage in an ongoing dialogue *between* the discrepant selves (Be Close/Don't Be Close). Here is the first exchange of that dialogue:

BE CLOSE: Just imagine the fun you could be having. You wouldn't have to put on an act for anybody anymore. You could just show people yourself and be able to do the things you really want to and not always submit to what everybody else wants you to do.

THERAPIST: Move to the other chair and speak from that side.

DON'T BE CLOSE: That sounds all well and good, but there's always the chance that they may not like who I really am. They may decide after I let them in that they don't want anything to do with me. They may be doing it because they just want something from me. And if I let them in, then they may feel like they're justified in coming to me. I don't think they really want to hear what I have to say.

As the dialogue proceeded along these lines for a few exchanges, a core discrepancy emerged. Barbara had a rational self who gave logical reasons why she should move closer to people, and a more emotional self who sought safety from being hurt. The rational self did not acknowledge the fear and hurt of the emotional self despite several clear statements of these feelings. The "Be Close" self did not provide any support for the other self when it expressed fears. At this early point, the dialogue lacked the necessary compassionate and understanding engagement that results in change. The "Don't Be Close" self seemed to realize this and said:

> "I'm not getting any support [uncomfortable laugh] and so I'm taking over. It's just not worth it. There's no point in it. If I can get through life just how I am that's fine. [rising voice] That's all I need."

The "Be Close" side responded that when the "Don't Be Close" side became stubborn like this, she felt "overpowered and drowned out." We concluded this session and reminded Barbara of her homework: to turn her assumptions about other people into hypotheses.

Session 2

Barbara reported that her mood had been somewhat better since our last session, but she also stated that she had "moody" days associated with asking her roommate to move out because she was sloppy and inconsiderate. The "moody" reaction was due to anticipation that the roommate would talk critically about her. This led to a discussion of her assumption that people do not like her. Again, we worked with her to turn the assumption into a hypothesis that could be checked out, and directed her attention toward gathering objective evidence about the hypothesis. We worked out with her how she would experiment with this hypothesis between sessions.

As we continued, she described how her older brother and sister had admitted to her that they did not like her. She became tearful and upset when she was talking about her sister, saying that her sister's rejection was particularly painful, and that even today it was difficult for her to let her sister into her life. This is a different kind of in-session marker, referred to as "unfinished business," in which an individual reveals the lingering presence of bad feelings toward a significant other person. Therefore, we did not return to the two-chair approach but set up an empty-chair experiment. In the empty-chair experiment, Barbara expressed feelings of hurt, anger, and jealousy toward her imagined older sister, and in doing so experienced some relief, but the session ended with this work still in process. (see Daldrup et al., 1988; Greenberg et al., 1993; and Greenberg & Safran, 1987, for extended discussions of working with unfinished business.)

Session 3

At the beginning of this session, Barbara reported that her depression was noticeably better this week and rated herself at a 3 (on 10-point scale), as opposed to an 8 for the first session. She also reported that she did approach some people that she ordinarily would not talk to, and that her interactions had gone reasonably well. We worked out experiments for her to try during the upcoming Christmas break.

We invited her to return to the two-chair experiment and to describe the sides of that dialogue in her own words. She called one side the "Giving" side who was willing to put things aside and give to other people. She called the other side the "Shy" side that holds back from people. The dialogue in the first session had identified the sides as "Be Close" and "Don't Be Close." We followed her new identification of the discrepant selves, since changes like these often mark shifts in the individual's perception and experience of the ambivalence. This session was pivotal. Barbara arrived at a new understanding of herself and the nature of her struggle. Therefore, we present an extended verbatim segment of that two-chair dialogue below:

GIVING SELF: You are no fun to be with. No one wants to be around you if you are going to just withdraw. You can't just sit around and do nothing. [Ironically, the tone of the Giving Self was more lecturing than giving toward the Shy Self.]

THERAPIST: Please move to the other chair and respond.

SHY SELF: I may withdraw, but I am successful in avoiding rejection and hurt.

THERAPIST: Tell her more about why you are shy.

SHY SELF: I'm shy because I want to shelter myself from rejection. Rejection is too painful.

THERAPIST: Change back.

GIVING SELF: Rejection is a part of life. Everyone is scared sometimes. To be shy is ridiculous.

THERAPIST: Move to the other chair and tell her what you want or need from her. [A move to elicit the *need* implicit in the fearful shyness]

SHY SELF: You are not supporting me . . . or helping me when you tell me that I am "ridiculous." It just makes me more shy. (*pause*) . . . I want to withdraw even more.

THERAPIST: Move back and respond to what you just heard.

GIVING SELF: (*softer tone*) I guess you're right. I need to be more like a big sister to you.

THERAPIST: (*remembering the empty-chair work with her older sister*) Move back to the Shy chair and tell her if the Giving Self reminds you of your sister.

SHY SELF: (*immediately making the connection that the Giving Self was behaving toward her just as her older sister had done*) Yes, that right . . . (*tearful emotions*). That's exactly what you do . . . you do treat me just like she did.

THERAPIST: Change and respond.

GIVING SELF: (*sticking to her theme*) I'm only doing it for your own good. If I did not push you, you would just withdraw from people and continue to be lonely and depressed. You cannot stay the way you are. You have to try harder.

THERAPIST: Move back.

SHY SELF: (*speaking in a much stronger and more grounded voice*) I know you push me to try to help me, but your current actions don't help. (*She now gets more specific about her needs.*) I need you to be my big sister who *encourages* good things in me, picks me up when I'm down, . . . to just be there.

THERAPIST: Change again.

GIVING SELF: (*capitulating some, but trying to hold on to the old position*) My role is to keep you from becoming unhappy. I am tired of seeing you unhappy. I am working to get you to do the things it will take for you to be happy.

THERAPIST: Please respond to that.

SHY SELF: (*continuing to find her own voice and strength*) Okay, your intent is fine . . . but I don't like your methods. It upsets me when you talk to me like that. I resent you for always putting me down.

THERAPIST: Change chairs again, please.

GIVING SELF: (*softening noticeably*) It isn't fair that I put you down like my older sister. I didn't realize I was doing that. I don't want to be like her.

The session ended with the Shy Self reiterating that she needed support rather than condemnation. The Giving Self responded by promising more support. As an experiment, Barbara was asked to notice any times that she spoke to her self as her critical older sister had done. At such times, the Shy Self was to remind her that she needed support instead.

Session 4

Barbara returned after a Christmas break of several weeks and reported that there had been changes in her outlook and that she thought more often of positive things and remembered negative things less. She estimated that her depression was down to 2 or 3 on a 10-point scale. She reported, "As long as I opened up to people, they seemed willing and interested in associating with me." She acknowledged that her belief that she would be rejected if she approached people could not be entirely correct, and that she was beginning to question that belief even more seriously than before. She had approached people she ordinarily would not approach and these interactions went reasonably well. To continue the CBT work, we discussed her criteria for a negative response from others. She experienced a negative response if the person gave a quick response and returned to his or her task. A more positive response was indicated by longer responses, or by questions about her from the other person. We agreed that she should observe and rate people's responses to her.

She described the "negative voice" as much weaker, and noted that she had been powerfully struck by the insight from the two-chair dialogue that she had been criticizing and rejecting herself just as her older sister had criticized and rejected her.

As a way to help her solidify these gains, we suggested that she return to the two-chair experiment. Again, there was a redefining of the two sides. The Giving Self was now redefined as the Negative Self, and the Shy Self was redefined as the Positive Self.

As she engaged in the two-chair dialogue she understood that she did not want to get rid of the Negative Self because it did provide a source of motivation, but she did want to tone it down. Then the dialogue moved to the "lecturing and nagging" that the Negative Self had refined into an art.

POSITIVE SELF: You don't make it any easier to accomplish what I need to accomplish (*voice tight*). In fact you make it a lot harder. I become anything but motivated. It makes me not really want to do anything . . . (*pause*) . . . It doesn't make me feel good at all. I am unhappy when you start nagging and criticizing me.

NEGATIVE SELF: Well . . . I only do it to keep you going . . . (*pause*) . . . Maybe it's not such a good way, but sometimes when you're pushed hard enough, you tend to work harder. Or something that you don't believe or somebody tells you can't do, you tend to work to show them . . . (*pause*) . . . I'm not really doing it to hurt you, but to help (*pause*) . . . but maybe it's not really helping.

Here we find the beginnings of a shift in posture, a questioning of whether the old position works. This questioning was followed by this exchange:

POSITIVE SELF: I need you to support me, and tell me I can do it and accomplish the things I want to . . . within reason of course . . . (*pause*) . . . but I need you to just be there for me. Stop tearing me down and telling me I can't do something . . . 'cause I'm almost at the point where if you tell me I can't do it, I just won't even try.

NEGATIVE SELF: Well, then, I can see where you're coming from. After being . . . after so many years, or whatever, being told you can't do something, you might actually start to believe it. I was trying to motivate you. In fact, I guess I've been wrong and I guess I need to change that. Actually, I know I do, 'cause I want to be there to help you. I don't want to bring you down.

This exchange demonstrated a shift in the dialogue. The Positive Self was able to state wants and needs in a voice that was increasingly clear and strong, while the Negative Self dropped its lecturing posture and listened to those needs. The Negative Self indicated a real intent to change her motivational style. The dialogue showed signs of honest resolution, with the Negative Self demonstrating that she understood that her position was harmful rather than helpful. Toward the end of the dialogue in this session, we found the Negative Self saying that she feels terrible:

NEGATIVE SELF: Terrible (small laugh).

THERAPIST: About yourself or about her?

NEGATIVE SELF: Feeling terrible about her. I'm upset with myself that I could ever do that to her.

THERAPIST: Tell her that.

NEGATIVE SELF: It wasn't right of me . . . I feel awful for that . . . I didn't realize . . . I'm angry with myself (very emotional).

THERAPIST: You're feeling a lot right now. Take your time with your feelings and then when you're ready, move to the other chair. (After a pause, Barbara moves to the other chair.)

POSITIVE SELF: You shouldn't be really angry with yourself. You were doing what you thought would help.

THERAPIST: (suggesting a sentence to say) And I just needed to tell you that.

POSITIVE SELF: Yeah, I just needed to let you know that what you were doing is . . . that the idea behind it [to point out all mistakes] was a good idea, but the way you were going about it just wasn't working. Just change the way you do it.

The two selves then negotiated how to interact with one another when there seemed to be a genuine need for some motivation. The Pos-

208 AMBIVALENCE IN PSYCHOTHERAPY

itive Self suggested that a reminder was acceptable as long as it did not become incessant. She was also clear that there was no intended harm, only an attempt to motivate. The Negative Self was grateful that the other side understood her motivation.

For CBT homework we worked out with her some motivational things she could say that would not be construed as harsh negative criticisms. She was to practice these new self-statements during the week.

Session 5

Barbara was given the BDI just before the therapy session and her score of 3 indicated that she was no longer depressed. She was pleased with her gains and reported that she was doing more with other people and feeling good about that. She had experimented with changing her level of interaction with others, and had found some interesting results. When she was quiet around her new roommate, the roommate was also quiet, but the more outgoing Barbara was, the more the roommate seemed to enjoy being around her. Barbara also listened for her "negative voice," and found that it had become more supportive.

In this session, Barbara did not seem to have any significant issues to discuss, so much of this session was spent consolidating the gains she had made thus far. When we inquired about her feelings toward her ex-boyfriend she shrugged her shoulders and said that she thought she was doing fine. However, a fleeting sadness crossed her face and her voice had a tinge of anger. To explore how resolved her feelings were, we interpreted these signs as another marker of "unfinished business" and asked her to have a conversation with her ex-boyfriend. We asked her to imagine him as if he was present in a chair in front of her. As she began to talk to him, she immediately became quite angry. She listed her complaints about him, and told him how frustrated he made her. Then, making a connection to earlier therapy work, she told him that he also did to her what her older sister had done—he brought out the negative in most situations. We continued to prompt her to make statements about her feelings toward him, and, in doing so, she expressed her feelings of hurt and broke into tears, expressing her feeling that he had not been fair. The tears continued as she told him that she had believed that he was her best friend and that she felt betrayed by him when he left her.

Because the end of the session was nearing, the therapist suggested that she say anything else she had to say and then say "good-bye." When confronted with saying good-bye, she found herself crying again and said that she did not think she could do that. She concluded by saying, "I don't want to let you go. I still care for you. I don't want to let you go." We had to conclude the experiment, though we were unclear about how resolved she truly was with this relationship.

Session 6

Barbara continued to show no signs of depression. She had followed up on her work from the previous session of letting go of the relationship with her boyfriend. During the week she had put pictures of him away, and felt as though she had put him in the past. This left her feeling good about herself, with occasional feelings of "emptiness." With experiential interventions, there can be an "incubation effect" where the experiment brings into high relief the full experience of the client and a new emotional understanding that leads to new behaviors and insights over time.

Barbara mentioned that she was not ready to date at this point. She also pointed out that she did not like to express her needs in a relationship because to do so was to risk being hurt. We focused on her belief that "If I express my needs, I'll get hurt." Once again, we suggested that she view this belief as a hypothesis rather than an assumption, and suggested that she try to do some small and relatively safe experiments with her roommate to test the hypothesis. Since she had been so creative in constructing earlier experiments, we left the details of the experiment to her.

There were overtones of the previous theme of wanting to get close to people and fearing to do so. Therefore, we invited her once again, to return to the two-chair dialogue to explore that ambivalence. This time the sides were identified as the Scared Self and the Wanting Self. In the two-chair experiment the Scared Self began by saying that things were going so well that she was afraid to ruin the gains she had made. She revealed that the therapists' suggestion about experimenting with her roommate made her apprehensive. She elaborated on the gains she had made and indicated that she was reluctant to chance anything that might jeopardize that.

The Wanting Self reminded her that she spent more time with people, but they were not yet her friends because she was still keeping them from knowing her. She said that there was a need to be cautious, but not this cautious.

The dialogue continued along these lines until the Scared Self told the Wanting Self how she felt toward her. The Scared Self said that she was not upset with her but that she needed something: "Make sure you don't push me into anything. Make sure you don't go too fast. I'm willing to try, but don't get too far ahead of me." The two selves discussed how they could monitor the pace of events while continuing to move ahead.

Although this two-chair dialogue had overtones of previous dialogues, there was a striking difference in the tone. Barbara was much gentler with herself in the dialogue, and there was a clear absence of the strong negative and critical stance that colored the first dialogue. This dialogue showed solid contact and understanding between the two selves. Barbara was aware of this change and very pleased with her progress. We agreed that this would be a good point to discontinue therapy. We set a time for a follow-up interview.

Follow-Up

A 2-month follow-up interview with Barbara revealed that she was doing quite well. While she reported occasional "down" days, she no longer experienced true depression. She reported that she now had many more friends than before, and was being more open with people than she had been before. She continued to listen to both "sides" and to try to tone down the Negative Side, and continued to think of trying new "experiments" that would help her test out some of her beliefs.

In a telephone interview a year after our last session, Barbara reported that her depression was no longer a problem. She continued to make changes in relationships and now felt good about the people in her life. She had also been dating someone new for most of the past year; they were engaged to be married at the end of her graduate studies. She was very positive and upbeat, and reported that she still occasionally used some of the strategies we discussed, including toning down her negative side and initiating experiments to test some of her beliefs.

Final Comment

The cotherapy effort, which consciously focused upon the use of two different therapeutic approaches, was a gratifying experience. This combination of therapies appears to work very well together. It assures that therapy focuses on both the cognitive structures and the accompanying emotional components. We are committed to the belief that experiential work will not bring about lasting change until and unless there are clear shifts in cognitive beliefs and structures. It does not require two therapists to accomplish the task, but we combined forces because we wanted to create a solid test of the usefulness of combining these two therapeutic approaches.

SUMMARY

In this chapter, we reviewed various ways that ambivalence work can be used along with other therapy approaches, with ambivalence work as a prelude to another treatment, or combined with another treatment. Two-chair work and MI can be combined and integrated as well.

Ambivalence work fits very well with both humanistic and CBT therapies. There has been less exploration of combining this work with psychoanalytic therapies, although we believe it can be done and has the potential for increasing the effectiveness of the therapy. We briefly discussed the potential of ambivalence work for medical noncompliance, and we concluded the chapter with an extended case example of the integration of ambivalence work and CBT.

Comparison among Theories of Resistance

PSYCHOANALYTIC THERAPY

What Changes Are Resisted?

1. Awareness of unconscious wishes and drives that would cause anxiety.
2. Changing repetitive and maladaptive interpersonal patterns.
3. Changing pathogenic beliefs and internal object representations.

What Behaviors Define the Presence of Resistance?

1. Behaviors that attempt to avoid painful awareness or insights and that are usually considered to be manifestations of ego mechanisms of defense (e.g., repression, denial, projection).
2. Continued engagement in long-term repetitive and maladaptive interpersonal patterns.

Why Is Resistance Occurring?

1. Anxiety reduction through avoidance of anxiety-generating insight into or awareness of one's unconscious drives and impulses.
2. *"Diablos conocidos"* (familiar devils): The security and predictability of the familiar.
3. Protection of a sense of stable identity by not changing.
4. Fear of change.
5. Unconscious pathogenic beliefs that maintain symptomatic behaviors.

6. Vicious cycles in which the person's internal object representations from early in life are confirmed by the way the person perceives and structures his or her world in the present.
7. Secondary gain in which the person receives benefit from the symptomatic behavior.

How Do Psychoanalytic Approaches Work with Resistance?

1. Therapist interpretations identify defensive avoidance/repetitive interpersonal patterns in and out of therapy.
2. Therapist interpretations link defensive avoidance/interpersonal enactments in the transference relationship to the client's early conflictual experiences.
3. The client's insight that the present defensive avoidance/interpersonal patterns are manifestations of earlier conflicts reduces the client's need to engage in these patterns.
4. The client undergoes a corrective emotional experience: when the psychoanalytic therapist does not respond to the enactments as the client expected, the client begins to question the need to engage in them and begins to change them.

COGNITIVE-BEHAVIORAL THERAPIES

What Changes Are Resisted?

1. Compliance with the procedures of CBT during the session.
2. Compliance with between-session homework assignments or experiments.
3. Changes in distorted thoughts, attitudes, beliefs, and schemas underlying symptomatic and resistant (noncompliant) behaviors.

What Behaviors Define the Presence of Resistance?

Any behaviors reflecting noncompliance with either in-session or between-session procedures, assignments, or experiments. Specific examples are listed in Table 2.5.

Why Is Resistance Occurring?

1. The therapist's use of inappropriate reinforcers, inadequate reinforcement contingencies for desired behaviors, reinforcement of behaviors that conflict with the goals of therapy, or setting standards for changed performance too high.

2. The client's faulty beliefs and assumptions and the schemas on which they are based.
3. Negative therapist attitudes or lack of skill.
4. The therapist's inadequate or incomplete evaluation of the case.
5. Client characteristics such as poor impulse control or rigidity.
6. Problems in the relationship between therapist and client.

How Do Cognitive-Behavioral Approaches Work with Resistance?

1. By changing the eliciting stimuli and reinforcers that maintain client noncompliant behaviors.
2. By analyzing and correcting external factors that may interfere with the client's compliance in therapy (e.g., by structuring less demanding homework assignments that the client is more likely to complete).
3. By helping clients to correct their dysfunctional thoughts and beliefs and modifying the schemas underlying their resistance and other related problem behaviors by using direct (persuasion) or indirect (collaboratively examining distorted thoughts) methods.

HUMANISTIC-EXPERIENTIAL THERAPIES

What Changes Are Resisted?

1. Awareness of experiences contrary to or discrepant from the current self-organization.
2. Contact with self.
3. Contact with and experience of the environment.

What Behaviors Define the Presence of Resistance?

1. Denials or distortions of experience that are incompatible with the perceived self.
2. Behaviors that indicate ambivalence, reflecting an internal conflict among aspects of the self.
3. Resistance of direct contact with the environment.
4. Being stuck in a particular stage of the gestalt cycle.

Why Is Resistance Occurring?

1. Perceptions that are inconsistent with the individual's view of his or her self-organization are threatening and kept out of awareness.
2. Ambivalence or internal conflict in which a part of self that wishes to

change is in conflict with a part that resists change, with the individual usually not aware of that second part.

How Do Humanistic-Experiential Approaches Work with Resistance in Clinical Practice?

1. Therapist attitudes toward the client convey safety and acceptance that allow the client to more easily become aware of threatening aspects of the self.
2. The client internalizes the therapist's accepting attitude toward threatening aspects of the self.
3. Experiments (e.g., two-chair dialogue) help clients become more aware of and integrate aspects of the self that have been out of awareness and that contribute to resistance.

FAMILY SYSTEMS THERAPIES

What Changes Are Resisted?

1. Changes in the structure and rules of the family.
2. Changes in the symptoms of one of the family members.

What Behaviors Define the Presence of Resistance?

1. Noncompliance.
2. Hostility.
3. Attempts to control the session.
4. Repetitive dysfunctional patterns of family interaction.

Why Is Resistance Occurring?

1. Maintenance of the status quo.
2. Fear of change.

How Do Family Therapists Work with Resistance in Clinical Practice?

1. Resistance is an obstacle to be avoided.
2. Therapist enters into the family system and challenges resistance.
3. Relabeling and reframing resistant behavior.
4. Employing paradoxical interventions.

REACTANCE THEORY

What Changes Are Resisted?

1. We resist attempts by others and by ourselves to limit our freedom.

What Behaviors Define the Presence of Resistance?

Behaviors are noncompliance with directives or oppositional behavior.

Why Is Resistance Occurring?

1. To reduce the motivational state of reactance.
2. To restore the freedoms that we perceive to be eliminated, limited, or threatened.

How Does Reactance Theory Work with Resistance in Clinical Practice?

While there is no specific therapeutic approach associated with reactance theory, it follows from the theory that directiveness on the part of the therapist will elicit reactance/resistance, while supportive/empathic interventions are more likely to elicit change.

CONSTRUCTIVIST THERAPIES

What Changes Are Resisted?

Changes resisted are those that relate to the self-system.

What Behaviors Define the Presence of Resistance?

Behaviors are not specified but are probably similar to those of other theories, especially humanistic-experiential ones.

Why Is Resistance Occurring?

Resistance to change in the self-system occurs because the status quo provides security and consistency and change threatens the integrity of the self.

How Does Constructivist Therapy Work with Resistance in Clinical Practice?

Constructivist therapists convey empathy and compassion for the person's desires not to change, respecting the reasons the person has for resisting change. They also invite the person to change at his or her pace, rather than trying to force change.

References

Alexander, F., & French, T. M. (1946). *Psychoanalytic therapy: Principles and applications.* New York: Ronald Press.

Amrhein, P. C., Miller, W. R., Yahne, C. E., Palmer, M., & Fulcher, L. (2003). Client commitment language during motivational interviewing predicts drug use outcome. *Journal of Consulting and Clinical Psychology, 71,* 862–878.

Anderson, C., & Stewart, S. (1983). *Mastering resistance: A practical guide to family therapy.* New York: Guilford Press.

Aponte, H. J., & Van Deusen, J. M. (1981). Structural family therapy. In A. S. Gurman & D. P. Kniskern (Eds.), *Handbook of family therapy.* New York: Brunner/Mazel.

Arkowitz, H. (1997). Integrative theories of therapy. In P. W. Wachtel & S. M. Messer (Eds.), *Theories of psychotherapy: Origins and evolution* (pp. 227–288). Washington, DC: American Psychological Association Press.

Arkowitz, H. (2002). An integrative approach to psychotherapy based on common processes of change. In J. Lebow (Ed.), *Comprehensive handbook of psychotherapy: Vol. 4. Integrative and eclectic therapies* (pp. 317–337). New York: Wiley.

Arkowitz, H., & Engle, D. (1995, April). *Working with resistance to change in psychotherapy.* Talk presented at the meetings of the Society for the Exploration of Psychotherapy Integration, New York.

Arkowitz, H., & Hannah, M. (1989). Cognitive, behavioral, and psychodynamic therapies: Converging or diverging pathways to change? In A. Freeman, K. Simon, L. Beutler, & H. Arkowitz (Eds.), *Comprehensive handbook of cognitive therapy* (pp. 143–167). New York: Plenum Press.

Arkowitz, H., & Westra, H. A. (2004). Integrating motivational interviewing and cognitive behavioral therapy in the treatment of depression and anxiety. *Journal of Cognitive Psychotherapy, 18,* 337–350.

Arnow, B. A., Manber, R., & Blasey, C. (2003). Therapeutic reactance as a predictor of outcome in the treatment of chronic depression. *Journal of Consulting and Clinical Psychology, 6,* 1025–1035.

Baker, K. D., Sullivan, H., & Marszalek, J. M. (2003). Therapeutic reactance in a depressed client sample: A comparison of two measures. *Assessment, 10,* 135–142.

Balint, M. (1968). *The basic fault.* London: Tavistock.

Barlow, D. (2002). *Anxiety and its disorders.* New York: Guilford Press.

Basch, M. F. (1982). Dynamic therapy and its frustrations. In P. L. Wachtel (Ed.), *Resistance: Psychodynamic and behavioral approaches* (pp. 3–24). New York: Plenum Press.

Bateson, G., Jackson, D. D., Haley, J., & Weakland, J. (1956). Toward a theory of schizophrenia. *Behavioral Sciences, 1,* 241–264.

Baucom, D. H., & Epstein, N. (1991). *Cognitive-behavioral marital therapy.* Philadelphia: Brunner/Mazel.

Beck, A. T., Freeman, A., & Associates. (1990). *Cognitive therapy of personality disorders.* New York: Guilford Press.

Beck, A. T., Rush, A. J., Shaw, B. F., & Emery, G. (1979). *Cognitive therapy of depression.* New York: Guilford Press.

Beck, A. T., & Weishaar, M. (1989). Cognitive therapy. In A. Freeman, K. M. Simon, L. E. Beutler, & H. Arkowitz (Eds.), *Comprehensive handbook of cognitive therapy* (pp. 21–36). New York: Plenum Press.

Beck, J. S. (1995). *Cognitive therapy: Basics and beyond.* New York: Guilford Press.

Beisser, A. R. (1970). The paradoxical theory of change. In J. Fagan & I. L. Shepherd (Eds.), *What is gestalt therapy?* (pp. 110–116). New York: Science & Behavior Books.

Berg, I. K., & Miller, S. D. (1992). *Working with the problem drinker: A solution-focused approach.* New York: Norton.

Beutler, L. E., Engle, D., Mohr, D., Daldrup, R. J., Bergan, J., Meredith, K., & Merry, R. (1991). Predictors of differential response to cognitive, experiential, and self-directed psychotherapeutic procedures. *Journal of Consulting and Clinical Psychology, 59,* 333–340.

Beutler, L. E., Machado, P. P., Engle, D., & Mohr, D. (1993). Differential patient x treatment maintenance of treatment effects among cognitive, experiential, and self-directed psychotherapies. *Journal of Psychotherapy Integration, 3,* 15–32.

Beutler, L. E., Mohr, D. C., Grawe, K., Engle, D., & McDonald, R. (1991). Looking for differential effects: Cross-cultural predictors of differential psychotherapy efficacy. *Journal of Psychotherapy Integration, 1,* 121–142.

Beutler, L. E., Moleiro, C., & Talebi, H. (2002). Resistance. In J. C. Norcross (Ed.), *Psychotherapy relationships that work* (pp. 129–144). New York: Oxford University Press.

Blatner, A. (1991). Role dynamics: A comprehensive theory of psychology. *Journal of Group Psychotherapy, Psychodrama and Sociometry, 44*, 33–40.

Blatner, A. (1995). Psychodramatic methods in psychotherapy. *Psychiatric Times, 12*, 321–330.

Blatt, S. J., & Ehrlich, S. (1982). Levels of resistance in the psychotherapeutic process. In P. L. Wachtel (Ed.), *Resistance: Psychodynamic and behavioral approaches* (pp. 69–92). New York: Plenum Press.

Botelho, R. (2004). *Motivational practice: Promoting healthy habits and self-care of chronic diseases.* New York: Motivate Healthy Habits.

Bowlby, J. (1969). *Attachment and loss: Vol. 1. Attachment.* London: Hogarth Press.

Bowlby, J. (1973). *Attachment and loss: Vol. 2. Separation.* London: Hogarth Press.

Brehm, J. W. (1966). *A theory of psychological reactance.* New York: Academic Press.

Brehm, S. S. (1976). *The application of social psychology to clinical practice.* New York: Halsted Press.

Brehm, S. S., & Brehm, J. W. (1981). *Psychological reactance: A theory of freedom and control.* New York: Academic Press.

Bromberg, P. M. (1998). *Standing in the spaces: Essays on clinical process, trauma and dissociation.* Hillsdale, NJ: Analytic Press.

Broussard, D. (1993). *Measuring reactance in a non-reactive way.* Unpublished doctoral dissertation, University of Arizona.

Brownell, K. D., Marlatt, G. A., Lichtenstein, E., & Wilson, G. T. (1986). Understanding and preventing relapse. *American Psychologist, 41*, 765–782.

Burke, B. (2002). *Motivational interviewing: A meta-analysis of controlled clinical trials.* Unpublished doctoral dissertation, University of Arizona.

Burke, B., Arkowitz, H., & Dunn, C. (2002). The effectiveness of motivational interviewing and its adaptations: What we know so far. In W. R. Miller & S. Rollnick, *Motivational interviewing: Preparing people to change (2nd ed., pp. 217–250). New York: Guilford Press.*

Burke, B., Arkowitz, H., & Menchola, M. (2003). The efficacy of motivational interviewing: A meta-analysis of controlled clinical trials. *Journal of Consulting and Clinical Psychology, 71*, 843–861.

Burns, D., & Nolen-Hoeksma, S. (1991). Coping styles, homework compliance, and the effectiveness of cognitive-behavior therapy. *Journal of Consulting and Clinical Psychology, 59*, 305–311.

Burns, D., & Nolen-Hoeksma, S. (1992). Therapeutic empathy and recovery from depression: A structural equation model. *Journal of Consulting and Clinical Psychology, 92*, 441–449.

Cavender, J., & Arkowitz, H. (1999). *A coding system for verbal indicators of resistance.* Unpublished manuscript, University of Arizona.

Chamberlain, P., Patterson, G., Reid, J., Kavanagh, K., & Forgatch, M. (1984). Observation of client resistance. *Behavior Therapy, 15*, 144–155.

Christensen, A., & Jacobson, N. S. (2000). *Reconcilable differences.* New York: Guilford Press.

Clarke, K. M., & Greenberg, L. S. (1986). Differential effects of a gestalt two-chair intervention and problem-solving in resolving decisional conflict. *Journal of Counseling Psychology, 33,* 11–15.

Connors, G. J., Walitzer, K. S., Dermen, K. H., et al. (2002). Preparing clients for alcoholism treatment: Effects on treatment participation and outcomes. *Consulting and Clinical Psychology, 70,* 1161–1169.

Daldrup, R. J., Beutler, L. E., Engle, D., & Greenberg, L. S. (1988). *Focused expressive psychotherapy: Freeing the overcontrolled patient.* New York: Guilford Press.

Daldrup, R. J., Engle, D., Holiman, M., & Beutler, L. E. (1994). Intensification and resolution of blocked affect in an experiential psychotherapy. *British Journal of Clinical Psychology, 33,* 129–141.

D'Amato, R. C., & Dean, R. S. (1988). Psychodrama research: Therapy and theory: A critical analysis of an arrested modality. *Psychology in the Schools, 25,* 305–314.

Davis, D., & Hollon, S. D. (1999). Reframing resistance and noncompliance in cognitive therapy. *Journal of Psychotherapy Integration, 9,* 33–56.

Davison, G. C., & Valins, S. (1969). Maintenance of self- and drug-attributed behavior change. *Journal of Personality and Social Psychology, 11,* 25–33.

Davison, G. C., Vogel, R. S., & Coffman, S. G. (1997). Think-aloud approaches to cognitive assessment and the articulated thoughts in simulated situations paradigm. *Journal of Consulting and Clinical Psychology, 65,* 950–958.

Davison, G. C., Williams, M. E., Nezami, E., Bice, T. L., & DeQuattro, V. L. (1991). Relaxation, reduction in angry articulated thoughts, and improvements in borderline hypertension and heart rate. *Journal of Behavioral Medicine, 14,* 453–468.

Davison, G. C., & Zighelboim, V. (1987). Irrational beliefs in the articulated thoughts of college students with social anxiety. *Journal of Rational Emotive Therapy, 5,* 238–254.

de Shazer, S. (1985). *Keys to solution in brief therapy.* New York: Norton.

de Shazer, S. (1988). *Clues: Investigating solutions in brief therapy.* New York: Norton.

de Shazer, S. (1990). Brief therapy. In J. K. Zeig & W. M. Munion (Eds.), *What is psychotherapy?: Contemporary perspectives* (pp. 278–282). San Francisco: Jossey-Bass.

de Shazer, S. (1991). *Putting difference to work.* New York: Norton.

de Shazer, S., Berg, I. K., Lipchik, E., Nunnally, E., Molnar, A., Gingerich, W., & Weiner-Davis, M. (1986). Brief therapy: Focused solution development. *Family Process, 25,* 207–221.

Detweiler, J. B., & Whisman, M. A. (1999). The role of homework assignments in cognitive therapy for depression: Potential methods for enhancing adherence. *Clinical Psychology: Science and Practice, 6,* 267–283.

Dewald, P. A. (1982). Psychoanalytic perspectives on resistance. In P. L. Wachtel (Ed.), *Resistance: Psychodynamic and behavioral approaches* (pp. 45–68). New York: Plenum Press.

DiMatteo, M. R. (1993). Expectations in the physician–patient relationship: Implications for patient adherence to medical treatment recommendations. In P. D. Blanck (Ed.), *Interpersonal expectations: Theory, research and applications* (pp. 296–315). New York: Cambridge University Press.

Dimatteo, M. R., & DiNicola, D. D. (1982). *Achieving patient compliance: The psychology of the medical practitioner's role.* New York: Pergamon Press.

DiMatteo, M. R., Lepper, H. S., & Croghan, T. W. (2000). Depression is a risk factor for noncompliance with medical treatment: Meta-analysis of the effects of anxiety and depression on patient adherence. *Archives of Internal Medicine, 160,* 2101–2107.

DiMatteo, M. R., Reiter, R. C., & Gambone, J. C. (1994). Enhancing medication adherence through communication and informed collaborative choice. *Health Communications, 6,* 253–265.

Dobson, K., & Shaw, B. F. (1995). Cognitive therapies in practice. In B. Bongar & L. E. Beutler (Eds.), *Comprehensive textbook of psychotherapy: Theory and practice* (pp. 159–172). New York: Oxford University Press.

Dollard, J., & Miller, N. E. (1950). *Personality and psychotherapy: An analysis in terms of learning, thinking, and culture.* New York: McGraw-Hill.

Dowd, E. T., Hughes, S. L., Brockbank, L., Halpain, D., Seibel, C., & Seibel, P. (1988). Compliance-based and defiance-based intervention strategies and psychological reactance in the treatment of free and unfree behavior. *Journal of Counseling Psychology, 35,* 370–376.

Dowd, E. T., Milne, C. R., & Wise, S. L. (1991). The Therapeutic Reactance Scale: A measure of psychological reactance. *Journal of Counseling and Development, 69,* 541–545.

Dowd, E. T., & Wallbrown, F. (1993). Motivational aspects of client reactance. *Journal of Counseling and Development, 71,* 533–538.

Dowd, E. T., Wallbrown, F., Sanders, D., & Yesenosky, J. M. (1994). Psychological reactance and its relationship to normal personality variables. *Cognitive Therapy and Research, 18,* 601–612.

Eagle, M. (1999). Why don't people change?: A psychoanalytic perspective. *Journal of Psychotherapy Integration, 9,* 3–33.

Elliott, R., Greenberg, L. S., & Lietaer, G. (2004). Research on experiential therapies. In M. J. Lambert (Ed.), *Bergin and Garfield's handbook of psychotherapy and behavior change* (5th ed., pp. 493–539). New York: Wiley.

Ellis, A. (1958). Rational psychotherapy. *Journal of General Psychotherapy, 59,* 35–49.

Ellis, A. (1962). *Reason and emotion in psychotherapy.* Secaucus, NJ: Citadel Press.

Ellis, A. (1994). *Reason and emotion in psychotherapy* (2nd ed.). New York: Birch Lane Press

Ellis, A. (2002). *Overcoming resistance: A rational emotive behavior therapy integrated approach* (2nd ed.). New York: Springer.

Engle, D., & Holiman (2002). A gestalt-experiential perspective on resistance. *Journal of Clinical Psychology/In Session: Psychotherapy in Practice, 58*, 175–183.

Fairbairn, W. R. D. (1952). *Psychoanalytic studies of the personality.* London: Tavistock Press.

Fiske, S. T., & Taylor, S. E. (1991). *Social cognition.* New York: McGraw-Hill.

Frank, J. D. (1978). *Effective ingredients of psychotherapy.* New York: Brunner/Mazel.

Freeman, A., Simon, K., Beutler, L., & Arkowitz, H. (Eds.). (1989). *Comprehensive handbook of cognitive therapy.* New York: Plenum Press.

Freud, S. (1958). Remembering, repeating and working-through. In J. Strachey (Ed. and Trans.), *The standard edition of the complete works of Sigmund Freud* (Vol. 12, pp. 145–156). London: Hogarth Press. (Original work published 1914)

Freud, S. (1959). Inhibitions, symptoms and anxiety. In J. Strachey (Ed. and Trans.), *The standard edition of the complete works of Sigmund Freud* (Vol. 20, pp. 75–175). London: Hogarth Press. (Original work published 1926)

Gann, M. K. (1999). *Assessing reactance in a clinical population with ATSS.* Unpublished doctoral dissertation, University of Southern California.

Gann, M. K., & Davison, G. C. (1999). *Cognitive assessment of reactance using the articulated thoughts in simulated situations paradigm.* Unpublished manuscript, University of Southern California.

Gingerich, W. J., & Eisengart, S. (2000). Solution-focused brief therapy: A review of outcome research. *Family Process, 39*, 477–498.

Gendlin, E. T. (1978). *Focusing.* New York: Bantam Books.

Gendlin, E. T. (1996). *Focusing-oriented psychotherapy: A manual of the experiential method.* New York: Guilford Press.

Gladding, S. T. (1995). *Family therapy: History, theory, and practice.* Upper Saddle River, NJ: Merrill Prentice Hall.

Goldfried, M. R. (1982). Resistance and clinical behavior therapy. In P. L. Wachtel (Ed.), *Resistance: Psychodynamic and behavioral approaches* (pp. 95–114). New York: Plenum Press.

Goldfried, M. R., & Davison, G. C. (1976). *Clinical behavior therapy.* New York: Holt, Rinehart & Winston.

Graff, H., & Luborsky, L. (1977). Long-term trends in transference and resistance: A report on a quantitative method applied to four psychoanalyses. *Journal of the American Psychoanalytic Association, 25*, 471–490.

Greenberg, L. S., & Clarke, K. M. (1979). Differential effects of the two-chair experiment and empathic reflection at a conflict marker. *Journal of Counseling Psychology, 26*, 1–8.

Greenberg, L. S., & Dompierre, L. (1981). The specific effects of gestalt two-chair dialogue on intrapsychic conflict in counseling. *Journal of Counseling Psychology, 28,* 288–296.

Greenberg, L. S., & Higgins, H. (1980). Effects of a two-chair dialogue on focusing and conflict resolution. *Journal of Counseling Psychology, 27,* 221–224.

Greenberg, L. S., Rice, L. N., & Elliott, R. (1993). *Facilitating emotional change: The moment-by-moment process.* New York: Guilford Press.

Greenberg, L. S., & Safran, J. D. (1987). *Emotion in psychotherapy.* New York: Guilford Press.

Greenberg, L. S., & Watson, J. C. (1998). Experiential therapy of depression: Differential effects of client-centered relationship conditions and process experiential interventions. *Psychotherapy Research, 8,* 210–224.

Greenberg, L. S., & Webster, M. (1982). Resolving decisional conflict by gestalt two-chair dialogues: Relating process to outcome. *Journal of Counseling Psychology, 29,* 468–477.

Haley, J. (1976). *Problem solving therapy.* San Francisco: Jossey-Bass.

Haynes, R. B., Taylor, D. W., & Sackett, D. L. (Eds.). (1979). *Compliance in health care.* Baltimore: Johns Hopkins University Press.

Heilizer, F. (1977). A review of theory and research on Miller's response competition (conflict) models. *Journal of General Psychology, 97,* 227–280.

Hermans, H. J. M. (1996). Voicing the self: From information processing to dialogical interchange. *Psychological Bulletin, 119,* 31–50.

Higgins, E. T. (1987). Self-discrepancy: A theory relating self and affect. *Psychological Review, 94,* 319–340.

Higgins, E. T. (1996). The "Self Digest": Self-knowledge serving self-regulatory functions. *Journal of Personality and Social Psychology, 71,* 1062–1073.

Higgins, E. T., Bond, R. T., Klein, R., & Strauman, T. (1986). Self-discrepancies and emotional vulnerability: How magnitude, accessibility, and type of discrepancy influence affect. *Journal of Personality and Social Psychology, 51,* 5–15.

Higgins, E. T., Klein, R., & Strauman, T. (1985). Self-concept discrepancy theory: A psychological model for distinguishing among different aspects of depression and anxiety. *Social Cognition, 3,* 51–76.

Hoffman, L. (1981). *Foundations of family therapy.* New York: Basic Books.

Honos-Webb, L., & Stiles, W. B. (1998). Reformulation of assimilation analysis in terms of voices. *Psychotherapy, 35,* 23–33.

Jacobson, N. S. (1992). Behavioral couple therapy: A new beginning. *Behavior Therapy, 23,* 493–506.

Jacobson, N. S., & Christensen, A. (1998). *Acceptance and change in couples therapy: A therapist's guide to transforming relationships.* New York: Norton.

Kazantzis, N., Deane, F. P., & Ronan, K. R. (2000). Assessing compliance with homework assignments: Review and recommendations for clinical practice. *Journal of Clinical Psychology, 60,* 627–641.

Kendall, P. C., Krain, A. L., & Henin, A. (2000). Cognitive-behavioral therapy. In A. E. Kazdin (Ed.), *Encyclopedia of psychology* (Vol. 2, pp. 323–324). Washington, DC: American Psychological Association.

Kepner, J. I. (1987). *Body process: A gestalt approach to working with the body in psychotherapy.* New York: Gardner Press.

Kihlstrom, J. F. (1987). The cognitive unconscious. *Science, 237,* 1445–1452.

Kipper, D. A., & Ritchie, T. D. (2003). The effectiveness of psychodramatic techniques. *Group Dynamics: Theory, Research and Practice, 7,* 13–25.

Laing, R. D. (1969). *The divided self.* New York: Pantheon Books.

Lambert, M., & Barley, D. E. (2002). Research summary on the therapeutic relationship and psychotherapy. In J. C. Norcross (Ed.), *Psychotherapy relationships that work* (pp. 17–36). New York: Oxford University Press.

Lazarus, A. A., & Fay, A. (1982). Resistance or rationalization?: A cognitive-behavioral perspective. In P. L. Wachtel (Ed.), *Resistance: Psychodynamic and behavioral approaches* (pp. 115–132). New York: Plenum Press.

Leahy, R. L. (2001). *Overcoming resistance in cognitive therapy.* New York: Guilford Press.

Lepper, M. R., Greene, D., & Nisbett, R. E. (1973). Undermining children's intrinsic interest with extrinsic reward: A test of the "overjustification" hypothesis. *Journal of Personality and Social Psychology, 28,* 129–137.

Lewis, T. F., & Osborn, C. J. (2004). Solution-focused counseling and motivational interviewing: A consideration of confluence. *Journal of Counseling and Development, 82,* 38–48.

Linehan, M. (1993). *Cognitive-behavioral treatment of borderline personality disorder.* New York: Guilford Press.

Littel, J. H., & Gurvin, H. (2002). Stages of change: A critique. *Behavior Modification, 26,* 223–273.

Loghman-Adham, M. (2003). Medication noncompliance in patients with chronic disease: Issues in dialysis and renal transplantation. *American Journal of Managed Care, 9,* 155–171.

Luborsky, L., Mintz, J., Auerbach, A., Cristoph, P., Backrach, H., Todd, T., Johnson, M., Cohen, M., & O' Brien, C. (1980). Predicting the outcome of psychotherapy: Findings of the Penn Psychotherapy Project. *Archives of General Psychiatry, 37,* 471–481.

Mahalik, J. R. (1994). Development of the Client Resistance Scale. *Journal of Counseling Psychology, 41,* 58–68.

Mahoney, M. J. (1991). *Human change processes: The scientific study of psychotherapy.* New York: Basic Books.

Mahoney, M. J. (2003). *Constructive psychotherapy: A practical guide.* New York: Guilford Press.

Mahoney, M. J., & Marquis, A. (2002). Integral constructivism and dynamic systems in psychotherapy processes. *Psychoanalytic Inquiry, 22,* 794–813.

Marks, I. (1992, November). *Behavior therapy as an aid to self-care.* Paper presented at the meeting of the Association for Advancement of Behavior Therapy, Boston, MA.

Markus, H., & Nurius, P. (1986). Possible selves. *American Psychologist, 42*, 954–969.

Marlatt, G. A., & Kaplan, B. (1972). Self-initiated attempts to change behavior: A study of New Year's resolutions. *Psychological Reports, 30*, 123–131.

Meichenbaum, D., & Gilmore, J. B. (1982). Resistance from a cognitive-behavioral perspective. In P. L. Wachtel (Ed.), *Resistance: Psychodynamic and behavioral approaches* (pp. 133–156). New York: Plenum Press.

Meichenbaum, D., & Turk, D. (1987). *Facilitating treatment adherence: A practitioner's guidebook.* New York: Plenum Press.

Messer, S. B. (1992). A critical examination of belief structures in integrative and eclectic psychotherapy. In J. Norcross & M. R. Goldfried (Eds.), *Handbook of psychotherapy integration* (pp. 130–168). New York: Basic Books.

Messer, S. B. (2002). A psychodynamic perspective on resistance in psychotherapy: Vive la resistance. *Journal of Clinical Psychology/In Session: Psychotherapy in Practice, 58*, 157–163.

Miller, S. D. (1994). The solution conspiracy: A mystery in three installments. *Journal of Systemic Therapies, 13*, 18–37.

Miller, W. R., Benefield, R. G., & Tonigan, J. S. (1993). Enhancing motivation for change in problem drinking: A controlled comparison of two therapist styles. *Journal of Consulting and Clinical Psychology, 61*, 455–461.

Miller, W. R., & Rollnick, S. (1991). *Motivational interviewing: Preparing people to change addictive behavior.* New York: Guilford Press.

Miller, W. R., & Rollnick, S. (2002). *Motivational interviewing: Preparing people for change* (2nd ed.). New York: Guilford Press.

Minuchin, S. (1974). *Families and family therapy.* Cambridge, MA: Harvard University Press.

Minuchin, S., & Fishman, H. C. (1981). *Family therapy techniques.* Cambridge, MA: Harvard University Press.

Mitchell, S. A. (1988). *Relational concepts in psychoanalysis.* Cambridge, MA: Harvard University Press.

Morgan, R., Luborsky, L., Crits-Christoph, P., Curtis, H., & Solomon, J. (1982). Predicting outcomes of psychotherapy by the Penn Helping Alliance rating method. *Archives of General Psychiatry, 37*, 471–481.

Neimeyer, R. A., & Mahoney, M. J. (1995). *Constructivism in psychotherapy.* Washington, DC: American Psychological Association Press.

Newman, C. F. (1994). Understanding client resistance: Methods for enhancing motivation to change. *Cognitive and Behavioral Practice, 1*, 47–69.

Newman, C. F. (2002). A cognitive perspective on resistance in psychotherapy. *Journal of Clinical Psychology, 58*, 165–174.

Nichols, M. P., & Schwartz, R. (2001). *Family therapy: Concepts and methods* (5th ed.). New York: Allyn & Bacon.

Norcross, J. C., & Goldfried, M. R. (Eds.). (1992). *Handbook of psychotherapy integration.* New York: Basic Books.

Norcross, J. C., & Prochaska, J. (1988). A study of eclectic (and integrative) views revisited. *Professional Psychology: Research and Practice, 19,* 170–174.

O'Hanlon, B. (2003). *A guide to inclusive therapy: 26 methods of respectful resistance dissolving therapy.* New York: Norton.

O'Hanlon, W. H., & Weiner-Davis, M. (1989). *In search of solution: A new direction in psychotherapy.* New York: Norton.

Orlinsky, D. E., Grawe, K., & Parks, B. K. (1994). Process and outcome in psychotherapy: Noch einmal. In A. E. Bergin & S. L. Garfield (Eds.), *Handbook of psychotherapy and behavior change* (4th ed., pp. 270–376). New York: Wiley.

Oyserman, D., & Markus, H. (1990). Possible selves in balance: Implications for delinquency. *Journal of Social Issues, 46,* 141–157.

Patterson, G., & Chamberlain, P. (1994). A functional analysis of resistance during parent training. *Clinical Psychology: Research and Practice, 1,* 53–70.

Patterson, G. R., & Forgatch, M. S. (1985). Therapist behavior as a determinant of client noncompliance: A paradox for the behavior modifier. *Journal of Consulting and Clinical Psychology, 53,* 846–851.

Patterson, T. (Ed.). (2002). *Comprehensive handbook of psychotherapy: Vol. 2. Cognitive-behavioral approaches.* New York: Wiley.

Perls, F., Hefferline, R., & Goodman, P. (1951). *Gestalt therapy.* New York: Julian Press.

Phillips, E. L. (1985). *Psychotherapy revised: New frontiers in research and practice.* Hillsdale, NJ: Erlbaum.

Polster, E. (1995). *A population of selves: A therapeutic exploration of personal identity.* San Francisco: Jossey-Bass.

Polster, E., & Polster, M. (1973). *Gestalt therapy integrated.* New York: Brunner/Mazel.

Prochaska, J. O., & Norcross, J. C. (2002). Stages of change. In J. C. Norcross (Ed.), *Psychotherapy relationships that work* (pp. 303–314). New York: Oxford University Press.

Prochaska, J. O., & Norcross, J. C. (2004a). *Systems of psychotherapy: A transtheoretical analysis* (5th ed.). New York: Wadsworth.

Prochaska, J. O., & Norcross, J. C. (2004b). Stages of change. *Psychotherapy: Theory, Research, Practice, and Training, 38,* 443–448.

Prochaska, J. O., & Prochaska, J. M. (1999). Why don't continents move?: Why don't people change? *Journal of Psychotherapy Integration, 9,* 83–102.

Prochaska, J. O., Rossi, J. S., & Wilcox, N. S. (1991). Change processes and psychotherapy outcome in integrative case research. *Journal of Psychotherapy Integration, 1,* 103–120.

Project MATCH Research Group. (1997). Matching alcoholism treatments to client heterogeneity: Project MATCH posttreatment drinking outcomes. *Journal of Studies on Alcohol, 58,* 7–29.

Resnicow, K., DiIorio, C., Soet, J. E., Borrelli, B., Ernst, D., Hecht, J., & Thevos, A. K. (2002). Motivational interviewing in medical and public health settings. In W. R. Miller & S. Rollnick, *Motivational interviewing: Preparing people for change* (2nd ed., pp. 251–269). New York: Guilford Press.

Rogers, C. R. (1951). *Client-centered therapy.* Boston: Houghton Mifflin.

Rogers, C. R. (1961). *On becoming a person.* Boston: Houghton Mifflin.

Rohrbaugh, M., Tennen, H., Press, S., & White, L. (1981). Compliance, defiance, and therapeutic paradox: Guidelines for strategic use of paradoxical interventions. *American Journal of Orthopsychiatry, 51,* 454–467.

Rollnick, S., Mason, P., & Butler, C. (1999). *Health behavior change: A guide for practitioners.* New York: Churchill Livingstone.

Sackett, D. L. (1976). Introduction. In D. L. Sackett & R. B. Haynes (Eds.), *Compliance with therapeutic regimens.* Baltimore: Johns Hopkins University Press.

Safran, J. D., & Greenberg, L. S. (1991). *Emotion, psychotherapy, and change.* New York: Guilford Press.

Salkovskis, P. M. (Eds.). (1996). *Frontiers of cognitive therapy.* New York: Guilford Press.

Schacter, D. L. (1995). Implicit memory: A new frontier for cognitive neuroscience. In M. Gazzaniga (Ed.), *The cognitive neurosciences* (pp. 815–824). Cambridge, MA: MIT Press.

Schaub, A. F., Steiner, A., & Vetter, W. (1993). Compliance to treatment. *Clinical and Experimental Hypertension, 15,* 1121–1130.

Schlenk, E. A., Dunbar-Jacob, J., & Engberg, S. (2004). Medication nonadherence among older adults: A review of strategies and interventions for improvement. *Journal of Gerontological Nursing, 30,* 33–43.

Schlesinger, H. J. (1982). Resistance as process. In P. L. Wachtel (Ed.), *Resistance: Psychodynamic and behavioral approaches* (pp. 25–44). New York: Plenum Press.

Schuller, R., Crits-Christoph, P., & Connolly, M. B. (1991). The Resistance Scale: Background and psychometric properties. *Psychoanalytic Psychology, 8,* 195–211.

Schwartz, G. E. (1991). The data are always friendly: A systems approach to psychotherapy integration. *Journal of Psychotherapy Integration, 1,* 43–54.

Searles, H. F. (1977). *Countertransference and related subjects: Selected papers.* New York: International Universities Press.

Shoham, V., Bootzin, R. R., Rohrbaugh, M. J., & Urry, H. (1996). Paradoxical versus relaxation treatment for insomnia: The moderating role of reactance. *Sleep Research, 24a,* 365.

Shoham, V., Trost, S. E., & Rohrbaugh, M. (2004). From state to trait and back again: Reactance theory goes clinical. In R. W. Wright, J. Greenberg, & S.

S. Brehm (Eds.), *Motivational analyses of social behavior: Building on Jack Brehm's contributions to psychology*. Mahwah, NJ: Erlbaum.

Shoham-Salomon, V., Avner, R., & Neeman, R. (1989). You're changed if you do and changed if you don't: Mechanisms underlying paradoxical interventions. *Journal of Consulting and Clinical Psychology, 57*, 590–598.

Skinner, B. F. (1938). *The behavior of organisms: An experimental analysis.* New York: Appleton-Century-Crofts.

Skinner, B. F. (1953). *Science and human behavior.* New York: Appleton- Century-Crofts.

Skinner, B. F. (1961). *Cumulative record.* New York: Appleton-Century-Crofts.

Stein, K. F., & Markus, H. R. (1994). The organization of the self: An alternative focus for psychopathology and behavior change. *Journal of Psychotherapy Integration, 4*, 317–353.

Stern, D. (1985). *The interpersonal world of the infant.* New York: Basic Books.

Stiles, W. B. (1997). Multiple voices in psychotherapy clients. *Journal of Psychotherapy Integration, 7*, 177–180.

Stone, H., & Stone, S. (1989). *Embracing ourselves: The voice dialogue manual.* Novato, CA: Nararaj.

Stone, H., & Stone, S. (1991). A professional point of view—The psychology of selves. Available at http://www. delos-inc.com/Reading_Room/Articles/4/4.html

Stone, H., & Winkelman, S. (1985). *Embracing ourselves.* Marina del Rey, CA: Devorss and Company.

Strauman, T. (1992). Self-guides, autobiographical memory, and anxiety and dysphoria: Toward a cognitive model of vulnerability to emotional distress. *Journal of Abnormal Psychology, 101*, 87–95.

Strean, H. (1990). *Resolving resistance in psychotherapy.* New York: Wiley.

Strupp, H. H., & Binder, J. L. (1984). *Psychotherapy in a new key.* New York: Basic Books.

Sullivan, H. S. (1947). *Conceptions of modern psychiatry.* New York: Norton.

Sullivan, H. S. (1953). *The interpersonal theory of psychiatry.* New York: Norton.

Sutton, S. (1996). Can "stages of change" provide guidance in the treatment of addictions?: A critical examination of Prochaska & DiClemente's model. In G. Edwards & C. Dare (Eds.), *Psychotherapy, psychological treatments, and the addictions* (pp. 189–205). Cambridge, UK: Cambridge University Press.

Swoboda, J. S., Dowd, E. T., & Wise, S. L. (1990). Reframing and restraining directives in the treatment of clinical depression. *Journal of Counseling Psychology, 37*, 254–260.

Taylor, C. B., Agras, S., Schneider, J. A., & Allen, R. A. (1983). Adherence to instructions to practice relaxation exercises. *Journal of Consulting and Clinical Psychology, 51*, 940–941.

Tennen, H., Rohrbaugh, M., Press, S., & White, L. (1981). Reactance theory and therapeutic paradox: A compliance–defiance model. *Psychotherapy: Theory, Research, and Practice, 18,* 14–22.

Treasure, J. L., Katzman, M., Schmidt, U., Troop, N., Todd, G., & de Silva, P. (1999). Engagement and outcome in the treatment of bulimia nervosa: First phase of a sequential design comparing motivation enhancement therapy and cognitive behavioural therapy. *Behaviour Research and Therapy, 37,* 405–418.

Truax, C. B. (1966). Reinforcement and nonreinforcement in Rogerian psychotherapy. *Journal of Abnormal Psychology, 71,* 1–9.

Van Eijken, M., Tsang, S., Wensing, M., de Smet, P. A., & Grol, R. P. (2003). Interventions to improve medication compliance in older patients living in the community: A systematic review of the literature. *Drugs and Aging, 20,* 229–240.

Van Hook, E., & Higgins, E. T. (1988). Self-related problems beyond the self-concept: Motivational consequences of discrepant self-guides. *Journal of Personality and Social Psychology, 55,* 625–633.

Vincent, P. (1971). Factors influencing patient noncompliance: A theoretical approach. *Nursing Research, 20,* 507–516.

Wachtel, P. L. (1982). Vicious circles: The self and the rhetoric of emerging and unfolding. *Contemporary Psychoanalysis, 18,* 259–273.

Wachtel, P. L. (1991). From eclecticism to synthesis: Toward a more seamless psychotherapeutic integration. *Journal of Psychotherapy Integration, 1,* 43–54.

Wachtel, P. L. (1993). *Therapeutic communication: Principles and effective practice.* New York: Guilford Press.

Walter, R. E., & Peller, J. D. (2000). *Recreating brief therapy: Preferences and possibilities.* New York: Norton.

Watzlawick, P., Weakland, J., & Fisch, R. (1974). *Change: Principles of problem formation and problem resolution.* New York: Norton.

Wegner, D. (1989). *White bears and other unwanted thoughts: Suppression, obsession, and the psychology of mental control.* New York: Guilford Press.

Weiss, J., Sampson, H., & the Mount Zion Psychotherapy Research Group. (1986). *The psychoanalytic process: Theory, clinical observations, and research.* New York: Guilford Press.

Westen, D., & Morrison, K. (2001). A multidimensional meta-analysis of treatments for depression, panic, and generalized anxiety disorder: An empirical examination of the status of empirically supported therapies. *Journal of Consulting and Clinical Psychology, 69,* 875–899.

Westra, H. A. (2004). Managing resistance in cognitive behavioral therapy: The application of motivational interviewing in mixed anxiety and depression. *Cognitive Behaviour Therapy, 33,* 161–175.

Westra, H. A., & Dozois, D. (2005). *Motivational interviewing as a prelude to group cognitive behavioral therapy for anxiety: A randomized pilot study.* Unpublished manuscript, York University, UK.

Westra, H. A., & Phoenix, E. (2003). Motivational enhancement therapy in two cases of anxiety disorder: New responses to treatment refractoriness. *Clinical Case Studies, 2,* 306–322.

White, J., Davison, G. C., Haaga, D. A., & White, K. (1992). Cognitive bias in the articulated thoughts of depressed and nondepressed psychiatric patients. *Journal of Nervous and Mental Disease, 180,* 77–81.

Wilson, G. T., & Schlam, T. R. (2004). The transtheoretical model and motivational interviewing in the treatment of eating and weight disorders. *Clinical Psychology Review, 24,* 361–368.

Winnicott, D. W. (1958). *Collected papers.* New York: Basic Books.

Winnicott, D. W. (1971). *Playing and reality.* London: Tavistock.

Wright, R. W., Greenberg, J., & Brehm, S. S. (Eds.). (2004). *Motivational analyses of social behavior: Building on Jack Brehm's contributions to psychology.* Mahwah, NJ: Erlbaum.

Young, J. E., Klosko, J. S., & Weishaar, M. E. (2003). *Schema therapy: A practitioner's guide.* New York: Guilford Press.

Zinker, J. (1977). *The creative process in gestalt therapy.* New York: Random House.

Zuckerman, M., DePaulo, B. M., & Rosenthal, R. (1986). Humans as deceivers and lie detectors. In P. D. Blanck, R. Buck, & R. Rosenthal (Eds.), *Nonverbal communication in the clinical context* (pp. 13–35). University Park: Pennsylvania State University Press.

Index

Unpredictability, 57–58
URICA. *See* University of Rhode Island
    Change Assessment Scale

V

Validation resistance, 29
Values, clarifying, 168–169
"Vicious cycles," 17
Victim resistance, 30

Voice dialogue, 82–84
Voices. *See also* Selves
    in two-chair dialogue, 117–120

W

Weight loss, 60–61

Z

Zinker's gestalt therapy, 85, 86, 87–88